I0101924

TOWDAH

A Cancer Survivor's Song Of Hope

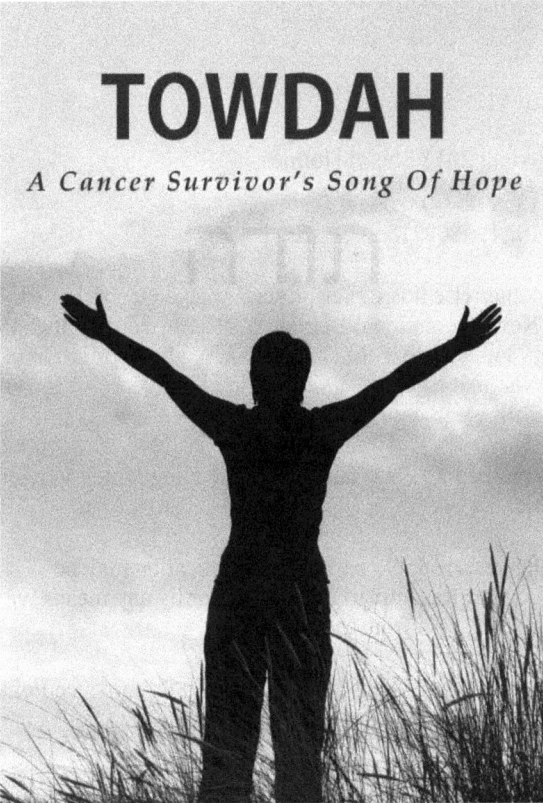

Sheryl Holmes

© Copyright 2012 Sheryl Holmes

ISBN-13: 978-1-938092-15-2
ISBN-10: 1938092155

Unless otherwise noted, Scriptures are taken from the Holy Bible, New International Version®, NIV®. Copyright © 1973, 1978, 1984, 2011 by Biblica, Inc.™ Used by permission of Zondervan. All rights reserved worldwide. www.zondervan.com.

Verses marked KJV are taken from the King James Version of the Bible.

All rights reserved. No part of this publication may be reproduced or transmitted in any form or by any means without written permission from the publisher.

Published by Pix-N-Pens Publishing, 130 Prominence Point Pkwy. #130-330, Canton, GA 30114, www.PixNPens.com

To order additional copies of this resource online, visit www.PixNPens.com.

Printed in the United States of America.

I dedicate these plain yet heartfelt words
to all who yearn to know
God will be there for them
when they are at their lowest.

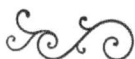

This is my story.

Purpose: Glorify my God

**"I will Praise God's name in song
and glorify him with thanksgiving."
Psalm 69:30**

Towdah is one Hebrew word for thanksgiving used in the Scriptures. This song is my offering of thanks given despite the suffering and difficult circumstances that I endured while dealing with cancer in my body. I lift up my hands in praise to my Abba Father and I thank Him for what He has done and for what He has not even yet done, but will do, because I trust Him. In and through my pain, I sing in agreement with my sisters of the past and say this: there is no other Rock like our God; He is my deliverer. He is the God who knew all I experienced and all I needed. I believed on the Words of my God to accomplish all that He said He would do; He was mindful of me in my humble state too. Mercy gushed over me every day. I repeatedly surrendered with offering *Towdah.* These offerings proclaim my song of thanksgiving to the Lord God, Jesus Christ, the one and only true and living God. I hope that He will find them a sweet sound in His ear.

It is my desire that **Towdah**: *A Cancer Survivor's Song of Hope* will display the sparkle of God in my life and the praise that I cannot keep to myself. Read my story and be encouraged, my friend.

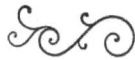

"Sacrifice thank offerings to God, fulfill your vows to the Most High; and call upon me in the day of trouble, I will deliver you, and you will honor me."

Psalm 50:14

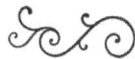

Contents

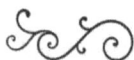

Offering One:
Love's Assurance

The sun beamed in like ripples of golden chiffon through the blinds. The sky was clear blue and a fresh breeze blew just enough to cause the leaves to rustle on the edge of the autumn season. Our walk across the parking lot a few moments earlier had been steeped in silence; hand in hand, we were in this together. Now, we waited. The clock ticked and the footsteps beyond the door became less frequent. Our eyes met and locked – yet neither of us dared to speak what was in our thoughts. Large in his frame and faithful in his devotion to me, David, my husband of twenty-five years was by my side.

The steps came closer and then stopped on the other side of the closed door. As the door cautiously opened, I saw it all on the steady face of my messenger. It was a forced smile as he held his hand out to me in greeting and he sat down just an arms-length away. He gently placed the file upon the desk and opened it.

My heart beat evenly, yet each rhythmic pound pressed against a weight a thousand times its own. My sweaty hands gripped the crisp white paper beneath me. Dread. Heavy dread. I just knew. I felt this exact way once before. Early August 1994, I sat in a waiting room with five months' worth of baby growth inside of me. My midwife couldn't get the right angle to find that tiny heartbeat – so an ultrasound was ordered immediately. Weakly I smiled as others passed by. Inside I was screaming. *Please God, don't let this be! You can do anything ... please let them find my baby's heartbeat.* Jumping up and down with earnest pleas, I was anything but calm. Because, just like this day, I just knew. Dread came. Unstoppable, dread settled in. This was it.

My messenger looked upon the sheet within the file that lay open on the desk and paused for just a second. Yet in that second, I suspected he was bracing and choosing his words carefully – pondering just how to say the words he had to say. He looked up at me with capital **C** compassion in his eyes and gently let the words slip off his tongue, "I regret to say that your tests revealed a malignant tumor." Simply and finally stated, "You have cancer."

After those words, I am not sure what else I really heard or even if I heard anything at all. It was as if a veil had been dropped during the interlude of the stage performance, and the dancers traveled through the dark forest off in the distance. Sound became fuzzy and dulled. I glanced toward David, and though our eyes met, I was unfocused and could only see the glazed outline of his familiar form as a silhouette against the sunlight still beaming through the blinds. I heard my dear husband let out a long and deep breath. Yet, I couldn't even be sure if I was still breathing. In fact, I am sure I was not. I was frozen – suspended as if above all concept of time. Again, I was jumping up and down in my heart, screaming … *"No, God. Let this not be true!"* I was numb.

Minutes added up to about a half an hour and my messenger peered at me with moist sorrow in his eyes, gently extending his hand. His hand was large, warm, and firm as he grasped mine in a hold that endearingly relayed, "I am so sorry." He exited the room. The door was left open, as he had offered us the private back door route out. As I slipped off the table, the crunching of the white paper underneath me crinkled with an unpleasant caustic sound. David stood with strength, only because he knew that's what I needed. He motioned me through the door, which led to a small, pocketed mini-foyer. Caught between the doctor's office and the crisp outdoors, we stood in silence for only a moment. Then, what we had been yearning to do since the files first hit the desktop, we did. We stood wrapped in each other's arms, falling into the well-known comforts of each other's bodies. My ear pressed firmly against his chest, listening to the beat of his heart, I sobbed. Dread had given way to a somber acceptance. We both took time to release the breaths we had suspended and they rushed out with abandon like a waterfall roaring over the cliff. Hand in hand, we opened the door and stepped into the brazen sunlight, neither knowing what lay ahead. But I assuredly knew that, along with God, my dear husband would be by my side always.

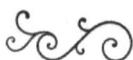

Offering Two:
The Telling

The *telling* in a family our size is always a production. The call goes out, as my husband bellows, roaming room-to-room like one calls "Olly, olly, oxen free!" at the end of a hide-n-go-seek game. He says, "Come to the living room – time for a family meeting!" Slowly, from all corners of the house and property come children of all ages. A few of them inquire with low-toned voices, "Is this a family beating or meeting?" Through the years, we have had plenty of reason to call the family together for chats for a variety of reasons. The children made their own code of discernment to know if it was a beating or a meeting. Any correcting or reprimanding or lecturing – well that's a beating for sure … all else, which wasn't much, falls into the category of meeting.

I had already found myself a place on one of the couches, trying to curl up and look as comfortable as possible, considering I was as uncomfortable in my own skin as could be. The children started filing in with that look of *uh-oh, what now* upon their faces. As I could see their apprehension, I recounted the many times we had gathered in a similar fashion. Each time I had gotten pregnant, we would gather and David would stand by my side, arm around my shoulder, and beamingly pronounce, "We have some news to tell you – Mom's going to have ANOTHER baby!" Kids would then jump up and down with a whooping and a hollering – 'YEAH!" Then the questions would come. As some of the kids got older, they knew the routine so well, that they refrained from whooping and hollering (the little kids did that), and smirked with uncertainty that seemed to ask – "really, mom, are you serious?" We did this a mere six times to the brood, once they were old enough to comprehend. In fact, David and I enjoyed their reactions so much – we, more than once, pretended to begin to make the "announcement" by just standing in that familiar stance with David's arm around me. He would start by saying, "Your mother and I have something to tell you …" We'd watch for their looks of momentary terror and excitement, and then David would say, "No, just kidding! But we do want to talk to you about your schoolwork …" Then the room would deflate like a popped balloon and the kids would hunker down into the couch and mumble, "Oh, this is a beating" and we would lovingly train them in the way they should be going.

But none of that was going to happen this time. As

the last child entered the full room, seeking the last squished spot on a couch, there was a definite heaviness and air of tension like fog rolling in on a cool evening. I tried my best to keep my composure as David spoke. "We have news to tell you, but it's not good. Mom has cancer." Suddenly I felt all nine pairs of eyes look at me, each like tiny probes piercing my heart in a most gentle way. What to say? What to do? No one knew. None of us had ever been here before. My faithful and steady husband continued in a very matter-of-fact way, explaining the type of cancer and the prognosis and the plan as far as we knew. We tried to convince them that we didn't have to worry because, after all, God is in control. That's what we had taught them – now we had to really show we were going to live it. Walk the talk.

A brief moment of silence ensued after David was finished with all the technical details. I asked if there were any questions. I got two responses that split off running in opposite directions. First, the one question no mom wants to have to try to answer from a dear young daughter. Her big round eyes urgently searched mine as she asked, "Mom, are you going to die?" My throat tightened, and my eyes filled. I told myself, *No – Sheryl, you must answer and you must not lose it!* I managed to say, as gently and convincingly as I could, "We are all going to die sometime. But the doctors are telling me that they are going to help me get better. So I am hoping that I won't be dying soon, or from this cancer, and that God will let me live a really long time." I smiled, trying not to look like I was forcing it, keeping my gaze upon the sweet daughter who was brave enough to wear her heart on her sleeve for me.

The second question came shortly after the first and totally re-directed the focus. This daughter said with eager delight, "If you lose your hair, can I pick out your wig?!" Night and Day. Heavy, Light. Yet both questions from the heart. One wanting the intimate *know* and the other wanting to be in the *doing* to help. What diversity comes with a large family! I laughed. And the laugh felt so good, as it released the ugly band of tension. More than one laughed as I said, "Sure!" There was immediate chatter as to what color hair I would have, how long it would be … and when this might happen. Moments from the telling of this not-good news, there was a jabbering of hope. I sat back, feeling a bit more comfortable in my skin as I watched the children slip into their familiar posturings as they each gave input as to what the wig choice would be. Conversation rumbled beneath *the look* that bridged over and above the din, between David and me. A knowing happiness was shared in the moment, a little light against the darkness.

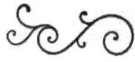

12

Offering Three:
Why Me?

Weeping in private became a regular thing for me those first few days after my diagnosis. The Bible describes hell as a place full of *weeping and gnashing of teeth* – a place we don't want to go. Yet, I felt like I was there. I was weeping and gnashing my teeth in the shower; heaving great spasmodic breaths, gasping for air in my voiceless cries. I was weeping and gnashing my teeth as I drooled and bit my pillowcase in the silent darkness of the night, when no one else was awake. I was weeping out of lack of understanding and gnashing out of frustration. *WHY ME, LORD?* I repeatedly wailed. Why me?

I promoted whole wheat bread to my friends before it was popular - always seeking out the most up-to-date healthy food to eat and preparing it for my family. (Just ask my kids - my creative experiments didn't always please the palates!). I didn't smoke. I didn't drink, except maybe a glass of wine or two a year; a six-pack of beer would last me an entire summer. I tried to take care of myself and had recently gone back to teaching dance; I had just finished taking a modern dance class, just for fun!

I was a good mom and wife. I worked hard at home, teaching the kids and running the household. I worked hard at church, volunteering time in countless areas of ministries. I was kind. I donated to the poor. I was honest. I've returned extra money given to me in change at retail stores. Yet, here I was. The one diagnosed with cancer. *Why me*, I asked. What about all those uncaring, overweight, smoking, drinking, lying, cheating, foul mouthed, greedy, no good doers! Why me? I was not happy and I was lashing out in my mind. Even now, as I write, I blush to think of my nasty thoughts. I felt like a little child in a full-throttled temper tantrum, screaming as I beat the pavement, *It's not fair!*

We've all been there. Those *why me* days are for every one of us. The baby is sick and running a fever, the washer is leaking, the stew is boiling over on the stove, the phone rings and as you go to answer it, the older child runs through the kitchen flailing a toy just out of reach of another weaker sibling, and inadvertently knocks over the coffee you had just poured in hopes for a caffeine boost to get through the day. And, we mutter, "Why me, Lord, why me? This is just not fair." Okay, okay … that's a little *why me*. With nine kids and living with both sets of parents for a time and a season, I have gone through a thousand and one, and more, of those little whimperings to the Lord.

But Lord, Cancer? This was a BIG 'Why ME?'! I was to the point of saying with exasperation, *How could you, Lord, allow this to happen to me!* Angry? Yes. Befuddled? Yes. Hurt? Yes. Indignant? Yes – ouch! Indignant before the Lord was not good. Colors of my character were coming out and I did not like the mix. Weeping and gnashing of teeth continued for days. Then I became weary.

Weariness gave up the gnashing. Weariness gave up the wailing, the heaving, the gasping, and the voiceless cries. Weariness birthed a stillness and a quietness before the Lord. I wept in my heart in silence as I lay in the darkness. In the morning, He came. He came through the voice of another brother who reminded me. Christ died for me.

That was it! I was asking the wrong question! It was like the sun breaking through the storm cloud. Strong, vibrant, focused, and with purpose. The question wasn't *why me, Lord?* The question I should've been asking was, *why not me!*

"But God demonstrates his own love for us in this: while we were still sinners, Christ died for us" (Romans 5:8). I am a sinner. I am saved; I had accepted God's free gift of salvation. Wasn't that enough? Is it enough? I had to decide. I could not find peace or resolution to this situation until I answered that question. Is salvation enough? Could I be content with just that? This was raw stuff. This was at the core of my being – gnawing deeper than ever. I felt like the whole of heaven was peering down, waiting to know my answer.

More questions came forth from my heart. Could I accept that God could do whatever he pleases with me? He could and would anyway. But, could I *accept* that? Could I, Sheryl, *believe* that God could do with me as he pleases just for His own purposes? I was at the fork of truth – my own, with the little **t,** and God's, with the big **T.**

I had to answer the questions that gnawed at me. After much grappling, I made up my mind to say, *yes! Yes, my Salvation in Jesus Christ is enough! No matter what, whether I live or whether I die, Jesus had already done more than enough for me. What more did I really need? Yes, Lord – "Why not me?"* It was clear I had to trust in knowing, "in all things God works for the good of those who love him, who have been called according to his purpose" (Romans 8:28). Was I being *called* for a purpose? Would it be good? Submitting with a willing heart, I uttered with resolve, *Okay Lord, Why not me?*

Yet, the struggle wasn't over and I grappled some more. The left side of my brain had reasoned out with logical understanding and I was good with my final decision to be in the place that says, *Why not me, Lord.* But, the right side of my brain was filling up with pictures, scenes, and images of Jesus in the Garden. As I lay upon my pillow in the dimly lit bedroom, I felt a warm tear trickle down the side of my cheek and ripple into the fibers of the fabric creating a wet pool against my face. I thought about Jesus in the Garden at Gethsemane, knowing His time was approaching to begin His journey to death. Images refracted from pictures and movies I had watched; Jesus went to pray. "Sorrowful and troubled" He went (Matthew 26:37-38). In my mind, I saw how He fell with his face to the ground and prayed (v. 39a). I pondered as I wept; the pool against my face was warmer and wider. Could Jesus have been asking, *why me?* Could Jesus have been struggling with obedience to His purpose? I imagined, with overwhelming depth of emotion, He collapsed face to the ground asking, "Father, if it is possible, may this cup be taken from me" (v. 39a). In my silent wondering, the tears now became a stream flowing, sopping my pillow. In my heart of hearts, I too fell to the ground and pleaded with God, *Please take this cup from me! Please?*

I felt close to my brother, Jesus. My eyes were opened to glimpse the depth of pain and anguish He must have felt during those moments of prayer. I was empathizing with Christ two thousand plus years later. Yet, time was irrelevant. Even in His anguishing pleas, Jesus gave it up to God. Could this have been like my weariness giving up the weeping and gnashing? "… yet not as I will, but as you will" (v. 39b).

Like the disciples with Jesus, who had fallen asleep, I had my husband next to me also asleep, his body rising and lowering with the even breath of a gentle snore. Though he was in this trial with me, close to my side, it was I who had to drink this cup of suffering, not he. It was me praying to God the Father, *take this cup from me.* Near drowning in my own puddle of silent flowing tears, I rolled onto my back, completely supine and vulnerable to my Father in heaven, and I prayed, *All right, me too, I agree. Not my will, but Yours Lord. Please use me as you see fit. Can you use me, even in this weak condition? Use me Lord. Use me Lord.* Sobbing ever so softly, peace filled me. The struggle ended. Yes, why not me; *Lord use me for your purposes.* A wave of calm and stillness came over me as I repeatedly I prayed, *use me Lord, I am yours*, until I drifted off to a deep sleep.

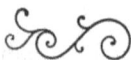

Offering Four:
Doable and Curable

Colorectal Cancer … Say that with correct and emphasized enunciation and it sounds like you are speaking the German language. The hard **C's** and **t** make it harsh and guttural. It is cacophonous to my ears – truly unpleasant. People would ask, "What kind of cancer do you have?" I knew they were just trying to be kind, yet, it was so embarrassing to have to tell. Who wants to talk about that area of their body? Nothing good happens there. Talk about the breast, that's life-nourishing and sensual; talk about the uterus, that's life-producing; talk about the throat, the liver, the tongue, the lung….just normal parts of the body. Let's talk about anything but the colon and the rectum!

I met with my oncologist. I liked her very much; her voice was gentle, yet she pulled no punches and was right to the point. I learned more about the colon and the rectum area of my body than I really ever wanted to know. Everything was just matter of fact. In the end, her final words to me were, "Sheryl, this is doable and curable – you're going to get through this!" Encouraged, I felt hopeful. Doable and Curable, would that be true? I thought about the Great Physician and my mind raced with urgent wonder. *Lord, is this doable and curable?* Rehearsing well-known Christian passages, I ran through, "All things are possible with God," (Mark 10:27b) and "Ask and it will be given to you" (Matthew 7:7a). I wondered how much of this outcome would be man and medicine and how much of this outcome would be God. Would I really make it through this? The questions and doubt were mounting. Fear gripped my every other thought. I had wished and prayed that my baby with the missing heartbeat would not be dead – again reciting in prayer, *"All things are possible with you, God."* But, my baby was dead – her heart was not jump started by the miracle healing hand of God. He did not choose that for His will. So how could I be certain that he would choose my treatment outcome to be doable and curable? Would it be His will for me to endure and live?

What choice did I have? Again, I was forced into thinking about some really right-to-the-core stuff; I searched my soul to discern what I truly believed. After twenty-two years of hearing His Word and studying and worshipping, why was this even a question in my mind? Could I trust God? Could I not trust God? Fear had a way of paralyzing my thoughts and actions. I was stuck. I couldn't proceed until I decided. I envisioned this trial as a very dark tunnel. I was not able to see anything beyond the opening configuration and that was labeled treatment. I did not know what that looked like, felt like, or would turn out to be like. I did not know what the other end of the tunnel looked like; the exit and what *I* would look like afterward. For a time, everything was an unknown.

In the movie *Fiddler on the Roof*, there are scenes where the father was caught, stuck in a thought, as he worked out a dilemma, and the camera pulled him out of the picture and re-focused him with a long and wide perspective of the issue at hand. That is how I felt, distant and set out of the picture of reality to think this dilemma through. On the one hand, I could trust in the words of my oncologist and hope she was right. On the other hand, I could trust in God, and no matter what, know I was in His will. Which is the more powerful? Then I chuckled a no-brainer chuckle and said, "duh!" Refocused, I came back into the picture, decision made.

I put my trust in God. I claimed the Scripture that the Lord God spoke to Joshua, "I will never leave you, nor forsake you" (Joshua 1:5b). As I faced this dark tunnel, I saw myself as the little child I was before my Father, God. Holding his hand, standing before the opening of treatment, I looked up at Him, with pleading in my eyes, and said, *You're really going to be with me, right?* And of course, in my heart, the Father squeezed my hand tighter and said, "Trust me, I said I would be." Later, I read and was comforted, "Be strong and courageous. Do not be terrified; do not be discouraged, for the Lord your God will be with you wherever you go" (Joshua 1:9).

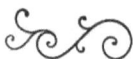

Offering Five:
Grace Abounds

The next few weeks brought me many appointments
with doctors and technicians. Everyone was gentle and
considerate, each taking care to keep my dignity intact.
However, each time, I melted inside. I was undressed. I
was poked and prodded for examination; I was filled with
gels and dyes of all colors and in all manners; drunk and
inserted. I was in a vulnerable place, exposed and not at all
in control or able to say *Enough!*

How could this feeling come from a woman who had
birthed ten children in all manners of doing: a la natural,
emergency style, and C-sectioned. I had exposed my
bottom end to hundreds of nurses, doctors, and technicians
over the years and I never cared who was in the room to
see before! The miracle of a life made the difference. This
time, I was not going to reap a beautiful outcome, a new
baby. This time I was seeking to destroy a deadly invader.
I wanted to curl up and hide in a corner of the darkest
closet I could find. I was humiliated, despite every discreet
effort of the people who so kindly were doing their jobs to
help me.

As I lay exposed upon white-papered table after

white-papered table, I began to sing. I had to shut out my circumstances to find my dignity. I was naked before strangers. I was naked before my God and I silently sang in my heart about how beautiful the Lord is, how I earnestly seek Him, and how I know that when He looks upon me, He pours out His grace in abundance. Grace, oh boy, I sure needed that! Singing to God was the only way I could disassociate myself from the painful and humiliating process of scans, procedures, and radiation. My God gracefully gave me the gift of peace and serenity and good humor to get through the beginning sections of that dark tunnel. My Father's hand tightly held mine. His eyes saw me and in my nakedness before Him, I felt no shame.

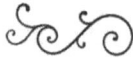

Offering Six:
A Slowed-Down Life

One morning, as I lazily wandered through the dining room, tired and subdued, my daughter came up to me and gave me one of her gentle squeeze hugs. With much contentment and a sigh, she said, "You're much nicer since you got cancer." BAM! Ouch! I was pierced. I was stunned like a deer caught in the headlights of an oncoming car. *Dare I ask her why*, I wondered. I paused. I asked.

She beamed up at me with a smile and said, "Cuz you don't yell so much anymore." BAM again! Double ouch! What does a mother say to that?

For the past seven years, I had prayed with my prayer partner at least once a week, sometimes more. A simple phone call on Wednesday mornings and we'd be off to the throne laying our needs before God. A persistent plea was for a slowed down pace of life, for I was always seemingly rushing around with my head cut off, often feeling overwhelmed with the circumstances of life. We began our prayer time together at her offering as we endured the days of my husband's ailing elderly father and his dementia issues while we all lived together under the same roof.

Daily, she called. I lived for those few minutes at the beginning of each day to have someone be with me in prayer, to boost me up for the day ahead. After my father-in-law's death, we continued in prayer, reducing to a once a week call. We prayed through the months of disruption as eleven of us lived in three rooms while we tore down half our home to re-build and re-model it. We prayed through ups and downs of the economy, skin-tight budget crunches, raising and teaching the kids, a winter of lice, and just the general efforts of living. We both lived full lives and we both often asked each other, *when will this life slow down?*

Well, here it was. I was truly and forcibly living a slowed-down life. Was this the answer to my persistent plea? Had this slower pace granted me the praise of my daughter? My heart was broken and I felt sick inside; *Oh Lord, did I really need to be brought here to acquire a more gentle spirit before my children?*

I admit I was a mother with a mission. I started with two children right from the start and never knew what it was like to have just one child. Then came three, and four … and with the numbers increasing, eventually up to nine, I became more organized and more vigilant with the duties of raising multiple children. I had pretty good control of my days and my children and I felt accomplished in most of my efforts with them. I pursued a happy home, and I laughed, and played, and allowed much clamor to give way to my kids' self-expressions. Art projects and building projects, pets and mess pervaded our home and property. Yet, I will admit, that at times, in order to keep order, I did bark and command, loudly; I needed no megaphone. My older boys lovingly called me Hitler-mom and my father in-law complimented me and told me I should've joined the military because I would've made a great Commanding Officer in the Army. I took some pride in those expressions about me because it portrayed a side of me that was in control and I liked that. Control meant order. And with nine children, multiple pets, and a household to maintain, order was a good thing. But, more than I'd like to admit, sometimes those barking commands came out of my mouth with the discordant sound of yelling, and without much love. Many times, I wanted ever so much to retract my words. But, I couldn't. So I often prayed, first with a sorrowful heart asking forgiveness for my sharpness with my kids and next I prayed with desire, *Lord help me to be gentle with my kids.*

So, some years later, with cancer attacking my colon, with radiation effects reaping havoc on my body, I was now granted the answer to my prayer: gentleness. How did it come? When did it come? When did she notice her mom was a nicer mom? I suspect it came when I arrived at the place of having no control, of having to give it all up to God. The order of my days was now not my priority. It was suddenly not that important. I recalled a newspaper clipping on my parent's refrigerator; "Every day you wake up above ground is a good day." I was beginning to *get* that. The order and 'to-do' lists of each day were not paramount to my functioning as a mom of nine children anymore. Did things get done? Yes. But they were done with less scurrying and much less barking. I had arrived and nestled into the niche of trying to see what was most important in my days and trying to appreciate my children more, each for who they were as individuals, rather than the brood of nine that were glommed together for so long under my wing.

Yes, my daughter was right. God had blessed me with the spirit of gentleness as I slowed down and relied more on Him for my each and every breath, above ground.

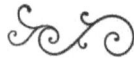

Offering Seven:
Lifted Up and Carried

The sun was shining beautifully and colored leaves now painted the sides of the road. I was on my way to one of my first radiation appointments, alone. My Aunt, also afflicted with cancer, had advised me to always have someone with me for my appointments for support. I had a good list of friends and family lined up to take me to all of the appointments, except for this one. I said to myself, *what's the big deal, I can do this, I don't even have any side effects yet.* So I proceeded out of the driveway and onto the familiar roads that led from my house to the local hospital where the radiation office resided. All was good.

Now radiation itself was not a big deal. It was a kind of Star Wars experience in a way, as I lay, exposed upon a table. Literal marker points were drawn on my body and these were aligned in a very specific way. The table was then raised up and pushed into a special machine, which beeped and flashed with lights that then fried me like a ray gun laser blaster! I felt nothing, aside from the momentary humiliation of having to bear my behind for the shooting. The technicians were great and always very considerate. The office was very homey; it was clear that they made every effort possible to make their patients feel comfortable.

Yet, the idea of radiation brought horrid and vivid images to my mind as I recalled a movie I had once watched where a man had been exposed to radiation from a bomb and he lay sick and shaking with delirium from fever, in a sterile room, dying from the inside out. It's amazing how images once entered into a brain never leave and can be recalled to the forefront of your thoughts in an instant, uninvited and without beckoning.

But, so far, physically, I felt fine. I got into the car. I selected a praise CD and was on my way home. Then it all hit. Emotions burst forth and my eyes filled with tears as I took in the words of the praise CD to combat the feelings of unrest. Every song was melting my heart. It was as if God Himself was cradling my heart in His hands and filling it with sweetness. I was in that dark tunnel called treatment, feebly stepping with hesitation and resistance, not wanting to go any further. Like a child, holding the Father's hand, I couldn't bear it anymore and I turned with anxious asking, *Pick me up, Daddy! I'm scared.* Each song on that praise CD worked its way into my fast beating heart and the tears flowed. I sobbed. I had to pull the car over at one point because the sobbing just came on with a vengeance. Where did this come from? Why now?

Just as images stuck in the brain come to the forefront in an instant, so too does God's Word that has been hidden in the heart through study and meditation. In between sobs, I realized my need for strength. I recalled bits of Psalm 28:7-9, "The Lord is my strength ... my heart trusts in him ... (*he*) is (*my*) shepherd and (*will*) carry (*me*)." Alone with God, I pulled myself together and reflected on the wisdom of my aunt. She was right. Moral support was a necessary element needed for these trips in the tunnel. Tomorrow would be another day and I was so looking forward to the company I would have.

Thirty days of radiation treatment with a little chemotherapy mixed in ensued. I was forever grateful for the ten people who accompanied me to my daily appointments. I was lovingly supported with great conversations, laughing, and quiet reflective moments on a bench by a duck pond. Even as the effects of radiation began to rip at my body, I was lifted up and carried by the care and servant hearts of the ones who chauffeured me to and fro. *They* were the arms of my Father, picking me up and carrying me in the scary moments in the tunnel each step of the way for six weeks.

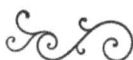

Offering Eight:
Comfort in the Leaning

I have known others to have cancer, go through the treatments, and get through it all. What I didn't know was the depth of pain and agony and hurt and fear and struggle they must have gone through. Until I had my own journey with cancer.

Nausea nagged like an annoying hangnail. It came in rolling, violent waves as certain pungent aromas drifted past; so bad that putting a sip of water to the lips was a feat beyond accomplishment at times – despite the orders to drink, drink, drink.

Sores and burns, like craters of festering wounds on the edge of the lip where soft wet mouth met the tough skin of the outer lip, splitting and bleeding; a sunburn down the throat and roof of the mouth wrinkled the skin; and a layer of scummy slime that would not leave the tongue caused everything to have a metallic non-taste to it – devastating to a person who loves food. More sores, in the armpits!

An itchy rash and a mild burn developed at the exit site of the radiation points; tender and uncomfortable, movement had to be at a minimum to keep it all at bay.

Like a tempest storm, blown in all directions, my intestines didn't know which way to go: diarrhea one day, constipation the next. Sitting on the porcelain throne was a wretched experience; labor pains were almost a second runner up to the kind of pain that it took to release myself. Hemorrhoids revealed themselves and I thought *I just might die.*

Discouragement started to build and I felt like a dormant volcano on the verge of erupting. Every emotion was just waiting for a reason to give way and explode.

I was totally IN the tunnel, there was no turning back, and forward seemed a slow creep, minute by minute – eons to pass an hour. I realized it was not an easy task to feel close to God when I wanted to curse Him for allowing the trial that afflicted me in such a hurt-filled way.

The opportunity arose for some comfort as I wearily stood in the kitchen one evening. David walked into the room and took me in his arms. Without words, I drew close to him, leaned against his chest and hugged him. We swayed gently to the music that wafted in from the other room and began an impromptu slow dance. Tears once again began to flow, streaming down my cheeks. No words. Emotions gave way with an ever so gentle explosion of sighs and tears. The music ended and we stopped swaying. I felt so loved, so uplifted, and strangely refreshed. Through the reach of my husband, God comforted me and took the urge to curse away. He blessed and I rejoiced and gave thanks for His provision of a most wonderfully loving husband who stood with me, swayed with me, and danced with me. He gave me what I needed – both of them. I was totally filled with the picture of Christ, the Shepherd, the one who cares and tends; "He tends his flock like a shepherd; He gathers the lambs in his arms and carries them close to his heart ..." (Isaiah 40:11).

Based upon Deuteronomy 33:27 are the words of an old Hymn:

> *"What have I to dread, what have I to fear, leaning on the everlasting arms? I have blessed peace with my Lord so near, leaning on the everlasting arms. Leaning, leaning, safe and secure from all alarms, leaning, leaning, leaning on the everlasting arms."*

And so I leaned, and I leaned hard! I leaned on God. I leaned on my husband. I leaned on my children. I leaned on my family and friends, and all who were near and dear. I think I was leaning on everybody I knew. Each in their own way represented for me the tireless arms of the Lord.

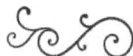

Offering Nine:
Prayers Offered in Faith

Prayer was an essential part of my traveling this journey through the darkness. With a weight of affliction as heavy as this was, I knew I had to pray, and pray long, and pray hard; and I did.

I recalled the words from James 5:14-15:

> "Is any one of you sick? He should call the elders of the church to pray over him and anoint him with oil in the name of the Lord. And the prayer offered in faith will make the sick person well; the Lord will raise him up. If he has sinned, he will be forgiven."

Claiming this Scripture, I called upon the Pastors and Elders of the church, and they came.

The children knew the Pastors and Elders were coming, so there was a hush in the house out of respect for the men and an understanding that this was a serious moment. As the men entered the living room, I sat with anticipation. I had called them here to pray for me – over me. I wanted the blessing of their faith-filled prayers. After a brief explanation of the procedure of this special prayer offering, four men lay their hands upon my back, my shoulder, and my knee. And in turn, they each offered up prayer for my healing. The warmth of their hands penetrated my countenance as if I was momentarily encased in a protective shell. I felt an energy hover about me. I wondered, *Is this the presence of the Holy Spirit?* I was anointed with oil on my head, a symbol of healing – hope. I was trusting in the faith of my Christian brothers. I was praying in agreement and desiring the full healing that they requested of the LORD. Knowing we each were powerless to accomplish what we asked for, we each knew God had the power to accomplish even more than we asked. This was an exercise of faith put to action. I believed. I was grateful for these men who took seriously the call to pray.

Prayer requests did not stop there. I wanted the full measure of the power of prayer because I wanted the full measure of complete healing. This was going to be a long haul, and I knew I couldn't do it alone. I decided to call upon the praying friends I had at my church and put out my requests on the prayer chain. Based upon my own prayers for people in the past, I always wished people would also follow-up with the answers to prayers. Mind made up, I resolved to keep a flow of requests and updates by way of the prayer chain until I was finished running through this tunnel.

What I did not count on was the network of God's people. Friends e-mailed me and encouraged me. They passed on my requests to at least three other local area churches. One friend living in New Mexico had her church praying there, as well as passing on my requests to a friend of hers in Germany. Missionary friends included me on their own e-mail newsletter, sent to hundreds of people up and down the East Coast. I had parents of a friend of mine in Missouri praying for me. And countless others I am sure, as people often said, "Oh, your e-mail was so pertinent, I sent it to a friend who needed to hear what you had to say …"

Schematics of airline traffic flow can be found on the internet, I once Googled that. What an incredible sight to see the red lines light up across the country; the world. I imagined that the network web of prayers offered up on my behalf must have looked similarly, only in vertical flow, directly upwards, parked at the feet of an incredibly big God. Each time I heard about someone passing on my prayer requests, I was awed. I was humbled.

I was lifted up.

God heard.

As my symptoms began to subside and I was healed

of my first round of treatment side effects, and as my tumor was shrinking, I was focused on Psalm 34.

> "I will extol the LORD at all times,
> His praise will always be on my lips,
> My soul will boast in the LORD;
> Let the afflicted hear and rejoice.
> Glorify the LORD with me; let us exalt His name together …
> I sought the LORD, and he answered me …
> The righteous cry out, and the LORD hears them;
> He delivers them from all their troubles.
> The LORD is close to the brokenhearted
> and saves those who are crushed in spirit."

I was praising Him for answered prayer! I was boasting in the LORD's goodness to me, despite my tiredness, weakness, and brokenness. I wanted everyone who prayed to know that God answered their righteous cries and He was delivering me!

Prayer requests and updates were my primary connection to family and friends. I was unable to attend church or any other activities for many months. My son often came home from church saying, "What do I tell people when they ask me how you are?"

I said, "Tell them I am being sustained by the LORD." There was nothing else I could say; that was the long and the short of it. I, plain and unknown Sheryl, the stay-at-home mom from Belchertown Massachusetts, was sustained by God's provision of the many faith-filled prayer warriors across the world; and His answer to their pleas.

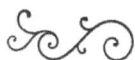

Offering Ten:
Compassion Overflow =
Boasting in God's Provision

Just like Paul expressed to the church in Philippi, I too yearned to express to the many, many people who partnered with me in this journey: "I thank my God every time I remember(ed) you. In all my prayers for all of you …" (Philippians 1:3).

Mail, money, and meals came in abundance. During the early weeks of my first treatment phase, a few cards came in the mail. I strung a bright pink ribbon across the double windows in my bedroom with anticipation and wondering if I could fill the string with cards as they came during this trial. Like not knowing God's network of prayer warriors, I did not know the far reach of the overflow of riches from people's hearts. Compassion abounded. The cards came, sometimes four or five in one day! I taped each one on the line of ribbon, and quite quickly filled it up, so I added another layer of ribbon. That line filled up with cards of all shapes and sizes; sweet endearing ones, inspirational ones, funny ones. My all time favorite was one that read: "Chemo sucks! But if it sucks the cancer right out of you, then Go Chemo!" I lay in bed at night and reflected on the goodness and kindness of my friends and family and even some from people I never even met. I surely felt loved. A few days would pass with no card, and I thought, *well, that's that*; so many well-wishers already, and my two lines of ribbon were sagging they were so full. I was delighted. But then, another one would arrive in the mail. By the end of the first phase of treatment, I had nearly one hundred cards layered and hung, on six strings of ribbons that ran across both sets of my double windows in the bedroom! In addition, I had children's handmade cards taped to my wall, and piled by my nightstand. My children were ceaseless encouragers; my cousin's daughter, and children from church also added to my piles. I was overwhelmed and I boasted in God's provision.

One movie that I totally enjoyed watching more than once, *Family Stone*, ends with a Christmas scene in which the family members receive a particular framed photo that just beats all, and ties the relationships of that family together; a pivotal moment that shows that love reigns. The mom in that scene gives a teary-eyed praise to the giver of the gift and said, "You done good!"

This past Christmas, I received a special gift from one of my sons that brought tears to my eyes and I too exclaimed with praise to him, "You done good, son!" He gave me a carefully crafted wooden box, purposefully made to hold all the cards I received from generous givers while I endured this trial. Today, the box is jammed tight and full with 257 cards and notes. I was, and continue to be, overwhelmed and I boasted in God's provision.

As if a card was not enough, several were often stuffed with money to help with my medical costs or meant for something special to treat us. More than once, those gifts came at just the right time when I was wondering of the Lord's provision, as we had no grocery money for the next week because I had to dole multiple-tens of extra dollars in unplanned-for appointments. The financial burden on one who has to go through such an ordeal is immense, even after health insurance! This too, was something I never realized about those who had gone before me and endured the cancer trial. I was ever so intrigued and grateful for one anonymous giver. Almost to the day, every couple of weeks for the entire duration of my suffering, I would receive a card signed, *God Bless You*, with various love offerings tucked inside: all types of gift cards for groceries, gasoline, household needs, a pizza night provision, or just a bit of cash to be used as I needed. If you are reading this, and it was you who was my anonymous giver, please know you touched my heart ever so deeply and I am forever thankful for your kindness to me and my family; may our Lord Jesus reward you for your giving in secret! From the twenty-dollar bill, to the five hundred, to the thirteen hundred dollar check, I was praising God for His moving among hearts to provide for our every need. Despite this trial in our lives, my steady working husband pushed on through his three jobs to provide, but even still, we were definitely coming up short. As we continued to pray, as bills piled on the desk, a few verging on "collection," friends and family moved with compassion, and by the Holy Spirit's nudging, provided. Once again, I was affirmed in my trusting God's Word, as Matthew 6:25 declares, "Therefore I tell you, do not worry about your life, what you will eat or drink; … is not life more important than food?" and later in verse 32, 33, & 34 "… your heavenly Father knows you need them. But seek first his kingdom and his righteousness and all these things will be given to you as well. Therefore do not worry about tomorrow …" God was, and is, my provider for all things that I need to be sustained. Again, I was overwhelmed and boasted in God's provision.

Literally, my family and I were also sustained by countless meals provided by both family and friends. For a year to the day, October 2010 to October 2011, we received at least one hundred and four meals, probably more if I counted the meals that my neighbor, my family, and my daughters and eldest son also lovingly made, as I lay on the couch dictating steps along the way. As my hands could not run under cold water or manipulate knives very safely, and as my nausea and fatigue plastered me to the couch more days than I liked, I was blessed by the hands of many, many people who prepared and labored to ensure that my family had good meals to eat. If you were one of those meal makers, I exuberantly say to you now, "Thank you, thank you, thank you!"

Slippers, nightgowns, lotions, plaques, and books, were supplied with loving intentions. Was I loved or what? Who was I to reap all this generosity? I often was rendered speechless. I often was found with a lump in my throat and tears welling up in my eyes. I am redundant! Let me make my boast in the Lord! He is Jehovah Jirah, My Provider!

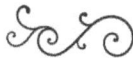

Offering Eleven:
Holding On

It had been weeks since I was able to attend a church service. My white cell count was up so I took the opportunity to go. It was like a breath of fresh air to my soul. So many friends to hug … so many friends to talk to – I was reveling in the chance to do it all. Singing was the best! I love to sing worship songs. The song, "You Never Let Go," spoke truth to me: God never lets go of us, whether we find ourselves in good times or bad times, God is always there for us. As I sang, I felt an *Amen* rise up in my heart. In this dark stretch of tunnel, my Father was still holding onto my hand assuring me he was not going to let go of me.

A friend sent me a card and gave me encouragement with words from Isaiah 43:2, "When you pass through the waters, I will be with you; and through the rivers, they shall not overflow you. When you walk through the fire, you shall not be burned, nor shall the flame scorch you." This passage reminded me that God was with those who persevered through the deep waters and the turbulent rivers and the hot fire and flame, and lived to tell about it. They were not consumed. I grabbed onto the hope in those words because I did not want to be consumed either. In faith, I knew I could stand, knowing my God would be with me in the same way. I held on.

My last week of the radiation and chemotherapy mix ended and the side effects came with a vengeance that culminated with horrendous hemorrhoids and I truly thought I'd never come out of the bathroom. Even through all four vaginal births, I never had hemorrhoids. I did not know what a Sitz bath was. Unfortunately, I knew all too well the last weeks of treatment. I read an entire book and took notes throughout, as I sat upon the Sitz! That's a lot of sitting and soothing. Mercifully, I was healed and I was not consumed.

Thanksgiving was fast approaching as I ended phase one of treatment. Many were fervently praying for me. I was pleading with God to heal me and end this pain. But, in my pain, I was reflecting on how I imagined it paled in comparison to the pain Jesus suffered on the cross for me. I didn't feel so desperate when I kept this vision of Jesus in focus. I found myself singing, "I will Bless Thee Oh Lord," over and over.

My hands were lifted up in honor and submission to my brother and Lord Jesus Christ, who died for me, a symbol of my lowly place before him, in adoration. My mouth couldn't help but follow with praise – for who He is; He is wonderful! He is my everything, my sustainer, my provider, my comforter, my strength, my peace … on and on. After praise, I couldn't help but fall right into thanks. I saw His character supplying me with all that I ever needed and I continued in thanks for my dear faithful husband, my sweet children, my servant-hearted family and friends, my soft pillow, my running hot water, food, good doctors, effective medicine, kind deeds, generous offerings, even yarn and knitting needles! If I kept on, I would never cease to find things to say thank-you for. But, was it really possible to bless the Lord? As I began this journey with cancer, I prayed, asking, *how can you use me in such a weak state?* Yet, I also prayed with acceptance of my situation, and said, *use me Lord as you see fit.* I knew that in the action of lifting my hands, praising His name, and thanking Him that I would make Him happy. In this, holding onto God's promises and Him still holding my hand, I could be used and I could bless my Lord.

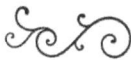

Offering Twelve:
100 Offers of Thanks

Traditions pervade the holiday season, and certainly help in holding a family close. A week or so before Thanksgiving, we all gather as a family and we pick out of a hat slips of paper that designate parts of the Thanksgiving dinner. Each one of us takes part in preparing the dinner, sharing in both the labor and joy of offering and being a part of the feast. It is a tense moment as we each see what part of the dinner we will have to make. Certain parts are vied for – the turkey, of course, being the prized slip of paper to obtain. However, girls usually liked the slip that read condiment tray, as that offers the opportunity to be creative and pattern the brightly colored veggies, pickles, and olives in a most attractive way. Nonetheless, we all take what we get and look forward to the day of eating. This year, I had a break from all of this preparation, as I had just finished phase one of treatment five days before Thanksgiving Day itself and I was too bedraggled to do much of anything.

Two movies are selected for this day because we really aren't football fans, so we rarely pay attention to that tradition of the season – commentators annoy me, and sports on TV are just boring. Just as my husband grew up never eating soup because his mother didn't like soup, my kids grew up never watching the football games, because their mother, me, didn't like commentators. But I love the old musicals and Disney movies. *Pollyanna* is a favorite, and so we watched it right after the morning viewing of the Macy's Thanksgiving Day Parade. The parade watching is always a delight for my husband because it has familial memory attached; David's maternal grandfather was an executive of Macy's in New York, and his office was used for a scene in the movie, *Miracle on 32nd Street,* which we watch in the evening, after dinner. We pause the movie each year to point out his mother's photograph that sat on the shelf behind the desk; strange connections cement the traditions.

The glad game is the gem in the movie *Pollyanna* that I love to pluck out from time to time and use on my children. This Thanksgiving, I was struggling greatly. On the one hand, I was in excruciating physical pain, and on the other hand, I was exceedingly thankful for having ended the six weeks of daily treatment. Determined to keep my focus in the positive, I numbered a large poster board one to one hundred, set it on the easel in our dining room, and challenged my family to fill it with one hundred things to be thankful for this year. I began it and listed about eleven things right away. Then I stepped back and retreated to the living room to rest.

The day proceeded with much flurry of activity, clanking of pots and pans and dishes being dirtied and washed in the kitchen; questions on cooking directions were sent my way. Laughter and memorized lines and comments resounded as the movies flashed by. The smell of the turkey cooking wafted through the house and all anticipated the flavors of the feast. I tried my best to think about eating, but truth be told, I was barely keeping down what little tidbits I snacked on. Even still, I was pleased and rested in the controlled chaos of my household. As the table was set and everyone sat, I slowly made my way over to the table with my donut pillow in hand. I carefully set it on the wooden chair, then eased my derriere upon it and smiled proudly. Despite my condition, my family had hung together and produced a lovely dinner. Tradition was good. My eyes glanced over to the poster board on the easel and my heart leapt for joy as I saw all one hundred spaces filled. Each in a variety of handwriting, there was tangible written thanksgiving offered. Bringing food to my lips was virtually impossible for me to stomach. I think I ate three spoonfuls of mashed potato and two of butternut squash, yet, I was full. I was full of Thanksgiving. This year, my family was that family gathered around the dining room table donned with turkey and the trimmings in the famous Norman Rockwell painting!

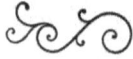

Offering Thirteen:
I Trust You, God

Blue and green attire breezed by me, in and out of the room, as I was being prepped for my third C-section. Number nine baby was about to enter the world. Suddenly, the intubation process had gone bad. I was aware, but unable to speak or even to breathe. My mind was fighting to tell my chest to rise and fill the lungs with air, but I could not move. It was like an elephant sat on my chest, holding me down. My eyes were still unable to open, yet, I could hear the panic level of rushing around me; a voice of authority was reprimanding a lower level assistant. I realized in a moment what was happening and I urgently prayed and called to God, *Please God, I am not ready to die – don't take me yet!*

Writing this eight years later, it's obvious that the anesthesiologist was successful in reversing the shut-down that they had induced, in time, and revived me to do an awake intubation. However, intubation was not a comfortable subject for me and not a process I was keen on having to endure again. Yet, as my first surgery approached, it was inevitable. I was anxious. I was worried. I was disconcerted. Searching for peace, I took the words from Philippians 4:6 & 7 and committed them to memory, trying to make them the fiber of my being so that I would truly believe them. "Do not be anxious about anything" (v.6a). How? "… but in everything, by prayer and petition, with thanksgiving, present your requests to God" (v.6b). I dashed to the computer, and presented my prayer requests, petitioning the intercession of as many as would take the time. I thanked Him for all that He had done in the tunnel for me. He was still my Father. I was still His child, gripping His hand tighter. Continually, I was repeating the question to my Father, *You're going to be there with me, right?* Verse 7: "And the peace of God, which transcends all understanding, will guard your hearts and your mind in Christ Jesus." I had to claim it. There was no rest for me if I didn't. So I did. No matter what, I again had to say, *I trust you, God.*

The night before my surgery, we stayed in a Best Western just a few blocks from the hospital. It was a crime really. It had been about six years since we had opportunity to stay in a hotel, alone, together, without kids. There was prep work to be done to clear out my system before the operation. I spent a good portion of the night in the bathroom. Thank goodness for the TV that entertained my dearly beloved. What a waste of a hundred and twenty dollars.

Even in the midst of trusting God, strange ideas passed through my mind as I was preparing for this major surgery. Removing a tumor, cutting out a section of my intestine, pulling another section of intestine to my abdominal surface and adhering an ileostomy was daunting and scary. *What if's* started playing out. What if I didn't make it? What did I want to say to my husband and children? Last words formed in my mind. In between runs to the bathroom, I set to writing notes to all nine children and my husband. Words of appreciation, love, and encouragement filled the papers. Accomplishing that, I was finally able to rest. Settled against my lover's chest, I drifted off to sleep and placed all my trust in Jesus.

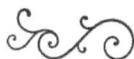

Offering Fourteen:
Life with Betty

Surgery was successful. Even though I had been methodically told about the operation and the ileostomy that would result, it still was a shock to look at my abdomen. I was sliced from the belly button down - a good six inches; swollen and very tender. A drain, like a straw, stuck out the left side of my lower abdomen. Just to the right of my belly button, IT was there. I groaned and looked away. IV's and wires and tubes and bags and soreness that rendered every movement feeling like a cat's claw ripping at my flesh, tearing and shredding it – burning with pain.

The good nurses came pleasantly, handling IT like it was nothing to be concerned about. They emptied IT for me, then showed me how to take care of the cleaning and emptying. Cheering myself on, I muttered in my head, *OK, Sheryl, you can do this – this is no problem, it's just a Ziploc with a major purpose and it won't be forever.* Bowel contents are no big deal. I remember one day, my husband and I sat down and tried to calculate how many diapers we might have changed through the years; at that point in time it was close to some ridiculous count of some thirteen thousand – and the first five children had cloth diapers! So what was a little Ziploc full of poop anyway?

The ride home was anything but comfortable despite the pain medication I was given before my departure from the hospital. Hunched over, I gripped the pillow firmly against my belly and I made my way with tiny baby steps to the house. I was greeted with smiles and twinkles in the eyes of my children. They ever so tentatively hugged me. Five days was a long time for mother to be gone from home.

The Lazy-Boy chair my brother had given me became my temporary niche. I slept in it for weeks as I could neither turn right or left without my abdomen feeling like it was going to pull off my body. It took about two weeks before I could even have enough strength to close the chair myself and get up without any help. This was a time I was glad for having many children to call upon for assistance; jokingly we laughed about the call, "Help I'm stuck and I can't get up!" – mimicking those commercials for help-call-button necklaces. Comedic moments were important!

It was also a funny moment when it occurred to me that I should name this bag. I had to refer to IT as something other than IT. So, Betty was born, Betty the Bag. It was easier to keep things light when I could say, "Excuse me, I have to take care of Betty now" or "Honey, can you help me with Betty?" Here again, a little dignity was restored and I felt a little more human.

Not so comedic were my experiences in the bathroom. My anger began to mount. I hated emptying the bag. The smell turned my stomach. The bloating of the bag from off-gases was embarrassing; I was sure everyone could notice it through my shirts. I began to wear big shirts and bulky sweaters to hide the problem. I was back to desperately asking, *Why me, Lord, why this! Hadn't I changed enough diapers?* Psalm 27:14 spoke to me: "Wait on the LORD, be of good courage, and he shall strengthen your heart; Wait I say, on the LORD" (KJV). Just as it is told, parenting isn't for the faint-hearted – so it's true for having an ileostomy. I surely needed a boost of courage and a strong heart to deal with the day in and day out, hour by hour, enduring. So I waited.

Showering was an interesting event. With the bag on, it was just hideous looking. Showering with it off, was, well … a dangerous event. It was bad enough that I had very little control of my bottom end since surgery. The muscles and trauma of the surgery often had me leaking much before I was able to get to the appropriate room to release myself. A naked stoma (the opening made by the small intestine brought to the surface of my outer skin) had a mind of its own. There was no control over when bowel contents were going to come out, or at what velocity either. Poop on the thigh was just a ghastly sight. I had to disassociate from this happening and I often talked to myself saying, *I did not do this! It was not me. It was the stoma – an entity all its own.* There. My dignity was restored.

Rashes persisted for several weeks until we found a base to the bag that didn't give me an allergic reaction. Changing, cleaning my skin, form fitting the base, securing the bag was a routine that was tiresome. But, David was my hero! He was my base form cutting expert; His large fingers dwarfed the tiny scissors used to precisely cut the base and work to fit it over my stoma. Here we were, caught in "the worst" category of our vows. Yet, I believe, it also was the ticket to the next level of love. It was easy to love each other when we were in the prime of our youth, beautiful and handsome, in each other's eyes. Now, scarred, and not so beautiful, I had a husband caring for me with the most servant of hearts and doing a most lowly job. This was deep love and devotion in action.

The emotion of it all was wearing on me. I felt heavy. I felt depressed. I was weak and felt I had become the very fabric of the furniture as I rested and waited for recovery from surgery. Having been through three C-sections, I was not totally ill-prepared for the recovery process. This however, was somehow different; so much more inner organ disruption. My back was compensating for my weak abs. I ached, front and back. I was bored. I watched way too many movies. Pain meds kept me from keeping a thought long enough to read effectively. It was too hot to knit. I was bored - totally bored. The kids ebbed and flowed with varying levels of cooperation; they too were tired of my non-activity. My tender-hearted young daughters often asked me, "Mom, when are you going to be done with this cancer stuff?" It was clear that they wanted their mommy back. I was lukewarm in my ability to praise God and I wondered if the kids were losing their grip on faith as well. Listlessly, I half-heartedly shot my prayers up and spoke more out of obedience than true belief that I would come through this ordeal. Depression was lurking in the doorway.

As time moved on, I did heal from the surgery and my ability to move around and get back into my bed did come. I recall the smoothness and softness of the sheets as I climbed into bed that first night. My bones sank willingly into the pad of the mattress and I let out an audible, *ahhhhh.* I smiled an uncontainable smile. It was a sweet night lying on my side, curled up next to my husband. Things were beginning to feel "right" again. I waited on the Lord. I felt a slow and steady drip of courage and strength being pushed through my heart. I thought, *Okay, maybe I can do this.*

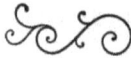

Offering Fifteen:
Love Never Fails

It was a snow-stormy day. My mother had left my younger siblings and me in the second floor apartment to go out and shovel the snow. All was well until I heard my mother crying out for me. I opened the door that led to the back stairwell and saw her crawling up the stairs. I was just five years old, and this was an amusing sight for me, so I began to laugh. Then, I noticed that she was crying and in obvious pain. Suddenly, the snowy afternoon took a serious turn. I stood there at the top of the stairs helpless, unable to pick her up and carry her, unable to do much of anything but look on with fear. Moms weren't supposed to need help like this; in my eyes, my mom could do everything. As she whimpered and gripped the upper stairs to pull her limp body up another stair, she directed me to get the phone. She knew she had to make it up to at least the top couple stairs to reach the telephone stretched to its fullest limit by the extra-long extension cord. Finally, as she was able to call for help, I felt relieved. This vivid memory in mind, I often wondered what my children were thinking and imagining as they watched me go through this difficult time.

Funny moments did occur, and always at my expense. Sitting at the breakfast table, just days after the installation of my ileostomy, it let loose with a gurgle, basically, a fart in a bag – totally out of my control. The eyes of my kids just became as wide as they could, aghast for a second then the next second gave way to an outburst of laughter. Except for the youngest of my girls, she was totally disgusted and shot me a look that was not very friendly or forgiving. As I excused myself from the table, I thought, *how can I get through this?*

A regular funny moment presented itself as they often watched me run, holding my bottom, over and around furniture and toys and laundry baskets in attempt to make-it to the bathroom. Yes, a funny sight to behold, unless you are the runner!

Walking across the parking lot on a short shopping outing, my girls chuckled along with me as my shoe flipped off, flying ten feet in front of us! This was neuropathy, a side effect from a chemo drug that caused me to lose the ability to scrunch my feet to grip my shoes. Sad but true, it was hilarious.

As side effects became more intense, I began to look and feel like my ailing in-laws that had since passed on. I leaked. I shuffled. I stumbled. Not really funny, but funny nonetheless. Losing control, not only of circumstances, but of my body was clearly evident. Viewed from the outside in, it was no doubt comical. To me, feeling from the inside out, I was devastated.

Even as I laughed at my mother, I remember it gave way to fear as I realized this was no joke. Donning wounds and bandages, ileostomy bags glued over a stoma – my body altered, and failing in energy and good memory recall, I was not the Mom that used to be here holding all things together. I could see the anxiousness in their eyes; the wondering if everything was going to be all right. Older children picked up the slack and worked to keep the household running; shopping, cooking, cleaning, laundry, tidying, schoolwork – over and over, day in and day out. Kind words, gathering and entertaining younger children so I could rest, spontaneous hugs that screamed unconditional love were given as offerings of commitment to me, their mother. The younger ones cuddled, caressed, and wrote me love notes that showed just how everything was going to be all right. God was working. The tables were turned, and my children wrote me notes covered with the Word to spur me on, and specifically explained that I didn't need to worry because *God was in Control*. Beyond their fear, they had a lifeline to Jesus. It was evident. Concerned for me, yes; questioning, probably; yet they were most definitely trusting in the One whom we had taught them about. Small-sized faith put into action was a lovely thing to witness! I was humbled by their focus on Him. I rejoiced with contentment, which bore peace in my heart. Unlike my memory of not being able to help my mother, being struck by fear, my children were strong and upheld and gave back to me the strength I needed in the Truths of Scripture.

Also with unconditional love, the mother I sought to help but couldn't, was now turned to me, looking on with the same grip of fear and helplessness. Life circumstances surely seemed all backwards and upside down. No mother should have to tend to a child with cancer. Cancer was supposed to be one of those old-people things to deal with. And too, a forty-seven-year-old daughter should be looking to help her almost seventy-year-old mother, not vice versa. Nonetheless, we had to deal with what God allowed. Tenderly, my mom came close and cared for me in many ways throughout, as a mother never stops caring and loving. I saw helplessness in her eyes and knew she just wanted to fix it and take away all my pain and trouble. Noble in its base and just in its desire, love never fails.

Walls that had built up in my family over the years began to break down. I was surprised. I was glad. Could it be that, in part, my suffering had a purpose in tearing down some of those walls? My sister stepped up to the plate and reached out with home-run-winning meals and special Auntie-times with my littlest girls. She e-mailed me with genuine concern, kept tabs on my treatments and my progress. One brother gave a recliner chair when it was needed. I lived in that chair for many weeks after both surgeries, and often thought of his kindness. The icing on the cake came as he walked into my hospital room, taking time for me. We had a one-on-one conversation for the first time in probably thirty five years. That was a gift from God for sure, another brick in the wall torn down.

My youngest brother, living an ocean away, came forward at the very end of my trip through the tunnel and gave a sweet monetary offering. Years had passed when we had little to do with each other, and changing that was not a priority for any of us. This life-threatening experience was like a low-level tremor, cracking the mortar and felling the bricks in the wall. Love prevailed – it did not fail. I was awed by the resiliency of love, even within a family that was always seemingly broken.

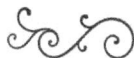

Offering Sixteen:
Mercy Poured and Grace Sealed

During the late and quiet hours of the night, we both needed comfort. This trial was bearing down on more than just me. When we took our marriage vows twenty-five years previous, we agreed to keep the bond for such difficult times as these that were now before us, for better, or for worse … in sickness, and in health. As young and naïve people in love we, of course, never imagined ourselves here. So it was each night as I attempted to fulfill union with my husband, I rolled away hiding my tears. I wanted to please and support my dear husband, as I knew he needed comfort too. Yet, I was in physical pain. Sorrow filled my soul.

Then, anger filled my soul. I stood weak, but vehemently, shaking my fist at my Father in Heaven, *Not this too! The one thing that has always been good in our marriage! Why are you taking this too?* I was mad. Passionate love was a blessing between us and we thanked God for it, often. I could even go so far as to say it was one of our strongest points in our marriage. Making opportunity for conceiving ten children was a delight; it was fun and it's obvious that God blessed us in our willingness and our pleasure to oblige.

Radiation took its toll on more than my entire digestive system. It had also attacked my feminine parts. As the physical pain increased, I resentfully sought out the doctors. As if having to talk about my colon and rectum and bowel behavior wasn't enough humble pie to eat, I now had to discuss my intimate life and my feminine parts and its pain and trouble with more professional strangers. Dignity was really at a low.

Apparently, radiation had honed in and penetrated my lower pelvic area and now, weeks later, effects were showing their ugly face. My vaginal walls had collapsed and adhered. Those adhesions had to be broken apart, not pleasant! Shooting, jabbing pain riveted through my body and I winced as sweat formed a bead on my brow. At the same appointment, it was also revealed that radiation had also annihilated my reproduction system and I was put into a forced menopause. Mentally, that was unsettling; I was fast-forwarded through the natural process of female aging. Disconcerted, I needed to adjust my self-image. The memory of that poor man in the movie, dying from the inside out, was once again thrown into vivid picture in my mind. *Was I dying too, from the inside out? I sure felt like I was.*

Wrapped and snuggled in each other's arms, we took

it on. The "or worse" and "in sickness" of our vows, was undeniably here. We embraced the horrid truth and we loved each other all the more. Patiently and gently, my lover tenderly spoke sweet and encouraging words to me and held me with an, "I'll never let you go" embrace. Over and over, the Lord God took us to the next level of love, deeper than the tangible now and stronger for it. Mercy was poured upon our marriage and our pledges were sealed by God's Grace.

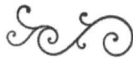

Offering Seventeen: Sister Ants

Ants are tiny creatures, yet they are strong. They are social insects and dependent upon each other to succeed. Each ant has a job to do, and together they work hard and build the colony. They accomplish this by constantly communicating with each other. Ant relationships are paramount to their triumphs.

I was expecting my family home from church any minute and I awaited the sound of the many swift footsteps clamoring on the back deck. Instead, I heard singing! The sound of female voices was growing louder and louder at the front door. Puzzled, I arose from my chair and opened the door. My jaw dropped and my mouth remained open in awestruck surprise. I found about twenty or so of my friends lined up and down the stony front walk, displaying all varieties and designs of pipe cleaner antennae on their heads! A myriad of voices were singing, "The ants go marching!" Smiling and giggling, the colony of sister ants came to say, "We missed you!" One dear friend came forward and placed a pair of pipe cleaner antennae on my head too. I couldn't say anything. I was utterly speechless. I knew why they had come and I was touched deeply in my heart. I couldn't attend the Ladies Retreat that past weekend because I was preparing and keeping my body from germs to maintain my best health before I started the second phase of chemotherapy treatments, scheduled for the next day. In twenty-two years I had only missed two retreats, and of all the years I wished and needed to go, it was this year. All I could muster to do was to go down the line of friends and hug each one. Each sister in Christ was special to me. Tears of joy, this time, not pain or hurt, trickled down my face. It was quite a scene to behold, I am sure, especially as we saw people on the street slow down, craning their necks to see what the commotion was about. It was a crazy moment. It was a fun moment. The vivid picture will never leave my memory! I bet there are not many, if any, in the world, that can say they had a colony of ants march in song to their front door to say we missed you and we are here to cheer you on as you start your next journey in the dark tunnel.

Nerves danced, as if in a mosh pit, in my stomach. I alighted the crown of antennae upon my head. I was ready. My friend, who volunteered to take me to the oncology office, arrived, also wearing her antennae. Yes, we were like young school girls, holding a secret and purposely being odd. We smiled wide grins as we drove on.

The office workers, nurses, and doctor looked on with

quiet enjoyment. I am sure they had seen silly things happen before. Humor had to be present from time to time to make this process bearable. I sat in the sterile recliner, ready to commence the six-month long race. The IV was in place, the pump was humming as it steadily dripped the drugs into my bloodstream. I was off. But, I was not alone. Twenty-plus sisters were with me in spirit. I was thankful. I was blessed. I closed my eyes and hummed, *The ants go marching ...* These sisters were paramount to my triumph through treatments.

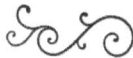

Offering Eighteen:
Rejoice in this Suffering?

For several days, the broken adhesions in my pelvis racked my insides in such a way that I had difficulty being in any other position than the classic fetal. I felt like a delicate flower and wanted to be placed on a high shelf away from everyone and everything. Curled up, I read Romans 5: 3-5,

"... but we also rejoice in our sufferings, because we know that suffering produces perseverance; perseverance, character; and character hope. And hope does not disappoint us, because God has poured out his love into our hearts by the Holy Spirit, whom he has given us."

Befuddled, I queried, *rejoice in our sufferings? Was that really possible? Who could do such a thing? Why should we do such a backwards act?* I got the part about suffering producing perseverance. I was suffering plenty and it did force me into persevering if I wanted to continue on with life. I understood that a persevering person would develop in character; it takes fortitude to carry on. It also spurs on a contrite heart, a willing vessel, and a vulnerable soul. Pain and suffering will produce a character of hope unless the one gives way to hopelessness, and denies the gifts of God, salvation through Jesus Christ, and the Comforter. So, I knew if I chose the gifts, and held them dear to my heart, I would not be disappointed. But, rejoice? How could I? I could not quite wrap my brain, or my heart, around that phrase.

Close on the heels of healing from the adhesions, I began the long haul of chemotherapy. I was anxious. Twelve treatment cycles equaled twenty-four weeks, which equaled six months. Six long months of more chemicals poured into my body. Yes, I had experienced the ugly effects of the chemo drug 5FU with radiation only a couple months previous, but I had not yet found out what the chemo drug Oxaliplatin would do. Would I lose my hair this time? Would I be sicker than before, or would I be able to stand up better against the poison that hid under the softened and necessary term: medicine? Unknowns filled me with fear. Lack of control surfaced again and I did not like this at all. I wanted to answer like the Sam in the Dr. Seuss book, *Green Eggs and Ham*, and turn my head and refuse it. No matter how it was presented, I did not, could not, would not, like this phase of the tunnel. No one could. I contemplated holistic approaches to healing cancer, but I could not find peace in them. Conventional methods are so ingrained in our societal understanding, that I reluctantly succumbed to the traditional medical model of treatment again, despite my inner being screaming, *No! Don't put the poison chemicals in this body!*

I was a classic model patient that reaped all the side effects as was predicted might happen by my oncologist. The 5FU, Oxaliplatin potion, was horrid. Nausea came - did that, knew that, dealt with that. My hair stayed – a silver lining! The cold sensitivities were minimal at first, but increased in intensity as time went on. I noticed it just barely four days into the first treatment cycle when I drank a glass of juice from the refrigerator. It was as if someone had put shards of glass in my cup because swallowing that gulp of liquid felt like someone scraped knives down my throat. I resisted the urge to run to a mirror and look for blood. Not long after that episode, I reached for meat in the freezer and surprisingly had to throw it quickly upon the counter as the cold pierced the ends of my fingertips like hundreds of tiny needles pricking my skin. I reactively cried, "Ouch!" Not thinking it through, I found myself exclaiming a loud *ouch* again after I tried to wash some vegetables in the sink – the cold water stabbed at me. I didn't quite understand what cold sensitivities would be

like when my doctor tried to explain them as a possible
side effect of the Oxaliplatin, but sadly, I knew too well
just a few days into the six-month race.

Nausea grabbed onto me with clenched fists and I
was prescribed Zophran. Burns rippled the skin on the roof
of my mouth and so I again took the prescribed miracle
mouthwash. My finger joints locked without any rhyme or
reason. Trickles of blood ran out my nose and I could
barely catch the small beaded puddle as it balanced on my
upper lip. Jolts of twanging nerve pains coupled with
muscle spasms in my back tied me in a knot. Pain knocked
me down into the Lazy-Boy with a dose of Oxycodone.
The burn and sting of the Neulasta shot nearly caused me
to jump out of my seat; this was an effort to perk up my
immune system and keep me able to fight off normal
germs. Payment was steep. I felt like I had the flu for
about three to four days after the shot was given. My body
ached and my muscles felt like bruises, I was hardly able
to keep my eyes open; I was so exhausted. Sleep was all I
wanted, but it was not mine to have unless I took a
sleeping aide at least for day one and two after the nasty
injection – insomnia was another side effect. The list of
gruesome effects seemed endless and only lessened
slightly at the end of my two week treatment cycle. The
couple of good days teased me. Sunday nights brought a

fight between me, myself, and I, as I tried to brush off depression. The crushing weight of anticipation settled and I had to push myself on through the tunnel and greet chemo-Monday and start the treatment cycle all over again. Rejoice in this suffering? I just couldn't do it.

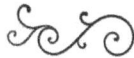

Offering Nineteen:
Rejoicing in My Sufferings!

Twenty-two years ago, I gave birth to premature twin boys. I went into labor and did not realize it until my water broke in my bath tub. My attempts to soothe and stop the contractions did not work. I was speedily transported via ambulance in the wee hours of a mid-summer morning, rushed into an emergency C-section, and found myself staring at two three-pound little babies struggling to live in the incubators at Baystate Medical Center in Springfield, MA. Overwhelmed was an understated way to describe me. During my first week at the hospital, a sleepless night gave me motivation to go visit my babies in the NICU (Neonatal Intensive Care) unit at 3 a.m. All was quiet. Sounds of soft chattering came from the direction of the nurses' station, rhythmic low beeps sounding from the machines that kept monitoring the babies' heart rates and oxygen levels. I sat in my wheelchair, staring longingly through the glass, wanting ever so much to hold my babies. Suddenly, I was aware of a man in black, standing next to me.

As I brought my gaze up to his face, I saw the white collar; he was a priest. His voice was calm and deep, as he asked me if he could pray over my babies. I immediately said yes. He prayed for God's watch over their lives. Then as suddenly as he appeared, he left my babies and me. I watched out of the corner of my eye as he continued on, standing over other incubators containing little lives struggling to survive. Much later, in retrospect, I thought, *how odd for a man to go around praying over babies at three in the morning.* Yet, in that lonely hour of that morning, God watered a seed in my heart.

My earliest recollections of God in my life came at my bedside when I was a little girl of four or five. My mother taught me to pray the famously recited bedtime prayer: "Now I lay me down to sleep, I pray the Lord, my soul to keep. If I should die before I wake, I pray the Lord my soul to take." Then I would thank God for my mom and my dad and my sister. In a little mind as mine, without a lot of training to understand, I was often confused about the "if I should die before I wake" part – it scared me a bit.

Where was this Lord going to take me anyway, I wondered. We went to church fairly regularly. It was a big, old, stone church with dark wood inside and deep tones of organ sounds filled the expansive space. I remember sitting next to my father, who seemed to be constantly looking at his watch, impatient to go somewhere. On the other side of me sat my mother, and she was always listening to the big voice speaking. I never understood what the man was saying. But I always felt serene and peaceful in that place. I loved the colored glass windows and the music.

A children's Bible was our bedtime story for a long time. I think my mother read the entire book to us. I was always happy to arrive at the end of the day, tucked into my pink sheets, and listen to my mom read the stories of Adam and Eve, Moses, and Jesus.

I began to have fond feelings for this God I was beginning to learn about. I liked him. I loved to play with the manger set under the Christmas tree, and at some point, I remember praying to God, asking him if he would make me be like Mary and bring Jesus back to earth again, so that I could be his mother. My small earnest desire was true in wanting to please this God, but I was extremely warped in my understanding.

Throughout my childhood, we went to a few different churches. I know I went to some of the Sunday school classes. But what I most remember was the spaghetti suppers, the punch and cookies, and the people all dressed up. I think I went on a youth retreat and there I remember making some fancy crafts. I made my first communion and had to memorize the Apostles creed. For a reward, my mother promised me a new Bible that had just recently come out, she said it was one that was more easily understood, called the Good News Bible. But I never received it. Even still, I felt an unexplainable peace inside me when I was in church. In my late teen years, I was the only one of my siblings who was willing to accompany my mother to church. I believe I had a decent set of morals because of the exposure. Many seeds were planted along the way, but not many seemed to take root. College and young adulthood came and I moved out and left the habit of going to church. My seeds were clearly dormant.

Almost a decade later, the prayer said in the wee hours of that morning watered the seeds that were planted in my childhood and an awakening began to grow. Those first three months of my baby sons' tiny lives brought lots of stress and worry and anxious wonder if they were going to live and be all right. In those wonderings, I realized that I had no control over their lives. I couldn't make everything better and I couldn't ensure their living. But someone had to have that control. I wondered if that God I had begun to learn a little about as a child was still operating. Was He the one that had control over all this life and death stuff? I offered up both suggestions and questions to my husband about the duty of bringing children to church. He recalled a small chapel down the street from our home, but didn't know if it was still open or not. We hemmed and hawed about whether we could give up our lazy Sunday mornings and the men's basketball league. At least we had to baptize these babies, we agreed on that. So we went to the chapel to get them baptized because it was the right thing to do.

Much watering went on as we continued attending the chapel down the street. One Sunday grew into a string of Sundays. Weeks, months, and years passed. The seeds grew, and we gained understanding and found the One who had control, who loved us, and died for us. That curious step through the doors in the fall of 1989 was the beginning of a new way of life for us. Twenty-two years later, we eagerly gave Sundays to worship God.

Cancer brought the routine of Sunday morning to a halt for me. My weak and sick body could not handle the people and all the germs, so I had to stay away. This was a major blow to my lifestyle. Loneliness set in. I missed my friends. I missed the worship, the singing, and the hearing of God's Word. Technology afforded my friend to tape the services, so I heard and saw the sermon the week after everyone else. And, I took to singing worship songs alone. Week after week, I sang to my Jesus.

It was a Sunday morning like any other, all the family had gone to church, and I sat in David's big recliner and began to sing the chorus, "Thank you Lord," a song about the Lord's readiness to freely give us salvation. Then, I read:

> " Sacrifice thank offerings to God, fulfill your vows to the Most High, and call upon me in the day of trouble; I will deliver you, and you will honor me … he who sacrifices thank offerings honors me, and he prepares the way so that I may show him the salvation of God" (Psalm 50:14-15, 23).

How long had I known that in my heart? How many days had I run and wasted by not living what I knew? I skimmed over the waters like a flat rock thrown in haphazard play. I needed to plunge deeper – to live deeper. Richer in salvation, I wanted to see more and know Him more.

Months ago, I searched for a way to get a grip on the calling in the book of Romans to rejoice in my sufferings. As I lifted up my single voice to God in song, I believe He blessed me with the answer to my seeking. I realized that the way to attaining joy and rejoicing in my sufferings was to have a heart of thanksgiving. Through the offering, the sacrifice of thanksgiving, I entered into relationship with God Himself. Singing and thanking the Lord for saving me, led me directly to praise. I could not help but praise

Jesus for the gift of salvation, for taking my sins, for healing my soul and making me complete in Him. In praise, He became really big and I became really small.

In my weak and humble state, I found salvation with grace and mercy meeting me there. I was feeling joy. I was rejoicing IN my sufferings! I was offering *Towdah*.

Despite cancer and all that comes with it, I was able to have a heart of thanksgiving and thank my Lord for all He was doing and all He would do in the days to come.

Cancer brought me out of the place of busy doing and into a place of being with the Lord. Cancer brought me low, made me slow, chopped my pride and control, and placed me with purpose, in a space and time for me to see Him more clearly. I found myself very alone before the Almighty that Sunday … offering thanks for the cancer. Yes, on May 22, 2011, I sat still and thanked God for my cancer.

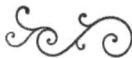

Offering Twenty:
Who am I? What do I Believe?

I think one of the first lessons in etiquette after please and thank you, must be the greeting of salutation: "Hello, how are you?"

"Oh, Hello, I'm fine, how about yourself?"

"Yes, I am fine too."

Fine; it's just such a trite word. I can never tell anything about anyone when they say they are fine. What does that mean? It's a cover up maybe … or an invitation to probe more … or a brush off? Who can tell? When I am the person being asked how I am, I need to take quick assessment of the situation and the person asking and determine within three seconds if this person really wants to know how I am, or are they just asking out of polite trained etiquette and is expecting the 'I'm fine' response. Hmmm … to tell, or not to tell, that was the constant question.

Years ago, I had a friend who also was tired of this trite expression and we decided to greet each other with an alternative salutation: "How goes it with your soul?" We just got right to the point. The temperature of the soul is really all that matters. Exchanging a smirk and a wink, we often would reply to each other with a line from a favorite old hymn, "Even so, it is well with my soul." The truth is that life, and situations in life, more often than not, doled out un-fine things. But, even still – all can be well with my soul. This is where I was, all the way through this tediously, unpleasant trial. I was very un-fine, more than very!

But, who wants to hear about the misery and the pain, over and over? Much like Job's friends, I am sure many of my supporters wanted only to move on. I related to Job in many ways and found myself curled up in a ball writhing with physical hurts and lack of understanding. I made conscientious effort to hold out and refuse to curse God for this trial. I really had much to praise God for, if I determined to look.

In the movie *One Night with the King*, Queen Esther was at a point where she had to decide whether to act on a difficult situation or not. She stood in deep thought and said, "Trials are meant (for us) to ask questions of ourselves." I was thoughtfully caught by that scene's message. Yes, I could agree. This trial definitely caused me to ask myself what I was really made of, and what did I really believe in. God allows things to happen. It is always His will. The Book of Amos (3:6) tells: "Does disaster come to a city unless the Lord has planned it?" Nothing is outside of God's plan. *Who am I? What do I believe?* Yes, I had to ask the questions of myself.

Balled up and feeling like Job, I meditated on the same favorite hymn:

> "Though Satan should buffet, though trials should come, let this blest assurance control, That Christ has regarded my helpless estate, and hath shed his own blood for my soul."

Who am I? I am one whose soul has been redeemed. What do I believe? I believe God had all this planned. "Even so, it is well with my soul." I have answered the questions this trial asked. "Whatever my lot, thou has taught me to say, it is well, it is well, with my soul."

I am surely more than just fine. How are you?

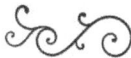

Offering Twenty-One: Jesus, My Only Plea

I knew it was coming. My brow was breaking a slight sweat, my mouth was watering, and I felt all clammy. I tried to swallow and tamp down the sick feeling, but I could not. I heaved the contents of my stomach. Not once, not twice, but more times than I could count. I began by running to the bathroom. I soon became too weak, so I brought a large bowl to my side as I literally lay on the floor, heaving and vomiting more than any one person could ever have done before. There was a stomach bug going around, at least that's what I heard, and that's what I assumed I was enduring in the beginning couple hours of being sick. Nine hours later, and barely a breath I could take in before I would be shuddering again with convulsions of my upper digestive system and cramps in my abdomen, likened to labor. This was not a normal stomach bug. I gave up and called my oncologist and she sent me directly to the local hospital ER.

At two thirty a.m., as I was wheeled on a stretcher to the ER X-ray, pumped with a dose of morphine to ease my pain, I weakly uttered, *Jesus please be with me.* I was depleted, completely drained. Jesus was my only plea. At that moment, I didn't really care if I lived or died, I only wanted Jesus with me.

I was diagnosed with a bowel obstruction and beginning pancreatitis, the reason for my wretched pain; oh how lovely - NOT. Food could not pass my lips, not even a drink for almost two days. The first sip of cranberry juice tasted like nectar from heaven when I was finally allowed to put something into my stomach. Thankfully, the obstruction cleared up and I did not need surgery. I needed to give my body a rest and so I remained in the hospital on observation and fluids for just about a week.

God answered me, and gave me Jesus during my hospital stay. In various ways, through the Holy Spirit prompts, Jesus was truly with me. Jesus was with me when a sweet sister brought me a book to encourage me. He was with me in the silent firm handhold of my husband. He was with me when a faithful brother came to pray over me. Love notes from my daughters poured Jesus' love out upon me. Another sister came with good humor and animated conversation and I felt Jesus tickling me and showering me with joy. Jesus came in the form of two dear friends over the phone, caressing me with caring words. A couple prayed with me and I felt the sustaining strength only given by Jesus. He was with me in the visits from my family of origin, reminding me that His love has always been there for me. In a one on one conversation with my blood brother, I felt the work of Jesus letting light into a bond that had been shut down for over thirty years. Jesus was certainly with me; in my moment of plea, the Father heard and answered. How awesome is that!

During the third night in the hospital, I lay in my bed, watching an amazing show of lightning bolts in the distance. Thunder growled and I was mesmerized. I began to sing, "Jesus, Lover of my Soul." This song sings praise to Jesus for lifting us out of troubled circumstance, setting us on a good path and the reactive desire to love Him and worship him no matter what; everything else can fail and fall but the one who loves Jesus will keep holding on.

I had sung that song many, many times, yet it was poignantly real to me that night. Especially in realizing that though I was sick, and weary, and left with no control over my situation, I still had my love for Jesus. As a believer in God, I had often questioned myself, wondering if things ever got really, really bad, would I have what it takes to stand firm in my faith in God? Now I was confident in answering that for myself. I clearly understood that only with Jesus could I stand in faith. I desired to worship Him, right to the very end, the very end of this hospital stay, this cancer journey, this life.

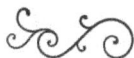

Offering Twenty Two:
Having it All

Twenty-six years previously, June 29, 1985, I was nervously nibbling saltines in my parent's living room, carefully sipping water so as not to drip anything on my white dress. It was a stormy summer evening and the electricity had just gone out. Luckily, we had planned a candlelight service, so no matter what, the wedding ceremony would go on. I didn't anticipate the level of emotion I would have as I walked down the aisle with my father by my side. I was a dancer. I was used to the stage and the lights. Performing was my game. Yet, I was trembling and I could hardly keep from crying as I steadily gazed upon my sweetheart at the end of the long walk through the middle of the church. Our vows were said, rings placed tenderly on each finger. The boom box blasted, *Celebrate*, by Kool and the Gang, as we were pronounced, "Mr. and Mrs. David Holmes." Joyously we linked arms and swiftly made our way out of the church that rainy June night. And celebrate we did! We fostered an invincible attitude as newlyweds. This life was great and we were gonna have it all!

David was beginning his career as a self-employed

contractor, I was dancing semi-professionally with plans to attend graduate school, and we had a cozy little apartment and a cat named Fuji. David's business had found a comfortable niche in a well-to-do neighborhood in Amherst, MA. I obtained my Master's degree and landed a nice job in Brattleboro, VT as a therapist. We built our own home; life was more than comfortable and we were on the road to having it all, just as we planned. Twins were on the way! On the brink of change, C.S. Lewis wrote in the *Chronicles of Narnia*, that, "Aslan was on the move."

Looking back, the conception of twins was the first hint of change coming; in Belchertown, God was on the move. Before I knew Him, God blessed me. I gave birth to twin boys and ended my professional-paid career. I went to church, met Jesus, and got baptized. God blessed again and I gave birth to number three son. The building boom crashed, David had no income, we sold our home and moved in with my parents. With mercy, God shifted David's career, we moved into an apartment, and He blessed me as I gave birth to our first daughter. Our second daughter was born dead, and with God's grace, we endured a devastating memorial service. God continued to bless and I birthed number four son, we moved again, and then again into David's parent's home. With laughter, God gave us our last son. David lost his job and God provided as he was hired by the state. Pouring out blessings of life, God delivered twin girls through me. David's mother suddenly died, and his father developed dementia, and he died a few years later. Blessing us again, I gave birth to our last daughter and I developed a blood disorder. We tore down half our home because it was falling in and lived for nine months in three rooms with nine children.

All the while I was home with my children, I home educated every one of them. I began to teach dance. One of our sons got married and we had a grandson enter our lives. Soon after, I was diagnosed with cancer. Yes, God was on the move and he drastically changed our lives.

On the eve of June 28, 2011, I lay close by my husband's side and recounted all we had endured in our marriage. Idle was not in the vocabulary to describe our lives together. We had been blessed beyond our haughty imaginings and we had it all – just not the *same all* we had originally set out to have, as invincible newlyweds. I wanted to forever stay cuddled against my husband's strong chest and savor the moment of reflection upon a full life. Momentary contentment filled my spirit. I was happy.

Tomorrow would be our twenty-sixth anniversary, but there would be no celebratory dinner. We would spend the day together at the hospital complex in Boston, preparing for and enduring yet another surgery. Despite the success of my first surgery, re-sectioning my intestine and installing an ileostomy – I was nervous for the reversal of the ileostomy. Would I make it through? Or was this my last day with my children and my last night with my husband? My mind reluctantly entertained the morbid thought. The check-list ran, even as I tried to savor the cuddle with my beloved: house in order, meals lined up, laundry done.

We arrived in Boston with about two hours to spare. It was a very warm sunny day. We did not speak much. There wasn't a whole lot to say. We shared quiet time on a bench watching the birds hop along the brick walkway as the city noise murmured in the background. David sipped a coffee and I was busy finishing the handwritten notes I had started the previous day - the *in-case notes* - so that I would have proclaimed my love and said my "thank-you" to each loved one again, in a tangible way. My mommy-heart was in overdrive. When time was up, we entered the familiar hospital corridors, on my way to be altered again. Change was continuing. The journey seemed endless.

Surgery was again successful and the next morning, in a drugged state, I was searching for Monica. I had high hopes that God would bless me again with her presence. Morning rounds had passed and I waited expectantly. During a light doze, I was awakened by a joyful singing of

"I'm Trading My Sorrows." A beaming smile came over my face as our eyes met, and I joined her in song.

Delighted and uplifted, I shared laughter with her. She had been my PCA (Personal Care Attendant) while I was in the hospital for the first surgery. Monica, a Jamaican Christian woman, was given to me as a gift from God as I endured the first painful walks around the unit, six months earlier. She was a light in my dark tunnel.

A five-day stay in a hospital two hours from home did not bring me any visitors. But God was on the move still. He was with me. My third day in the hospital, Josette was given to me. She was gentle in spirit and spoke with a thick accent; she was from Haiti. With a strong arm, she led me on my first painful walks around the unit this time. She sang me a song she had written in Creole and translated later to English. It was a song telling about how Jesus is always with us, and that he never leaves us. Blessed beyond my asking, she was God's messenger.

Day four arrived, and I was weary of the hospital scene. PCAs must gather and talk in their break room, because, as I heard the singing, I just knew word must have gotten out that I was waiting on God. No kidding, Lynnta, also from Haiti, came boldly in my room singing, "Lord, I lift Your Name on High," and I gleefully joined in. Smirking, she changed tunes and sang, "Shine Jesus

Shine," and I lifted my voice up with hers. We laughed. I was tickled by the Holy Spirit Who was so alive in such a place. Who would have expected or believed, that in a large public hospital in the middle of the capital city of Massachusetts, I would have three PCAs singing me praise songs with no care as to who was listening. I was comforted through my pain. I was visited daily by these sisters the Lord. I was encouraged because of three women who heeded the call. I was not alone. Even in the hospital, I had it all. I had the "all" that God had planned for me.

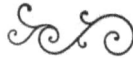

Offering Twenty Three:
A Friend Lays Down an Omelet

"Betty-the-bag" was history! She was not missed one bit. Though scarred and altered, I was so glad to have my body back. My digestive system had to be treated as if I was a newborn – liquids, to pureed food, to soft food, and eventually to a varied diet as I could handle it. The bowel obstruction had interrupted my chemotherapy cycles. I was glad for the break, even though healing from abdominal surgery for the second time in a six-month period was no joyous picnic.

Chemotherapy treatments resumed and though I had a break from the chemical invasion, my body reacted quite fiercely with side effects. My fragile digestive tract suffered most violently and I was forced into an eighteen-hour fast and back to a liquid diet because any food I ingested reaped havoc on my intestines. In addition to the usual nausea and cold sensitivities, I was weakened by hunger. My parched mouth barely allowed any liquid past my lips. I hit another low dip in the tunnel and I was feeling very alone in my journey, food wasn't even my friend – no comfort there.

Several days into this low dip, the phone rang. The

voice on the other end of the line surprised me. It was a brother in the Lord I had known nearly fifteen years, but not one who ever called me on the phone. Curiously, I listened. He said, "I just have to tell you …"

This man had just made himself an omelet for breakfast and was sitting down to his computer to check his e-mail, coffee in hand. As he raised the steamy bite of omelet to his mouth, he was in the middle of reading my prayer request about my inability to eat. He said he heard the Holy Spirit prompt him to stop, not eat his omelet, and to throw it away. Knowing this brother, I was stunned. This was a man who enjoyed his food immensely.

He continued, "What?" He himself was not sure if he had heard the urging correctly and so he paused. But then he described a feeling of true conviction. He had heard perfectly, and under a compulsion not his own, he threw the entire freshly made omelet in the trash. With confidence, this brother declared, "The Holy Spirit wanted me to share in your suffering today."

I was speechless. The tears welled up in my eyes and I could barely speak, telling him, "I do not know what to say."

This brother, another chosen messenger of the Lord, said, "I only shared this with you to encourage you … to let you know that the Holy Spirit is working and that you are prayed for." The phone call ended there.

I stood amazed. God's work was so much bigger than my despair. Paraphrased Scripture says that there is no greater love than the love displayed by a friend laying down his life for yours (John 15:13). This day, I had a brother lay down his omelet, his comfort, his nourishment, for me.

How great was that? He chose to suffer in hunger alongside me, from a distance. What an awesome picture of Jesus Christ, the kingly brother who gave his life for mine. How people go through fiery trials without God and the fellowship of His people, I will never know!

Astonished and comforted, I was uplifted and carried through the rest of the day feeling extremely loved, by my friend, and by my God.

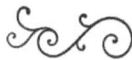

Offering Twenty Four:
Focus on the Unseen

Over the past decade, my husband has labored multiple hours remodeling and fixing up our very old house. Yet, the money was spent, with nothing left to completely finish the kitchen and bathroom. The bathtub has been the same water-stained tub for the past forty years, the sink is a decrepit '70s-style basin donning the gold speckled countertop. The floor is chipped tile that covers a spongy and partly rotted floor base. It is the sore of our homestead. Public bathrooms are more appealing than my own in-house convenience. A fresh coat of paint and bright towels try their best to re-direct the focus. The one popper of the room is a collage of all the children's bathtub baby pictures. Filling one of the photo slots is my handwritten copy of a portion of Psalm 139. My sensitive digestive system had me re-reading this Psalm repeatedly as I sat in pain and agony. "All the days ordained for me were written in your book before one of them came to be (v. 15)."

I exclaimed with some disdain, *Really Lord! This day was ordained for me? This pain-filled day was appointed for me?* With exasperation and tears, I cried, *Why?* I dared to question the Lord's motive and plan. Who was I anyway? Could I do that?

After a pause, I realized something profound. *Wow Lord! You planned this ahead … way ahead … before I was even born.* I could not even fit that idea in my head. I pondered this at a point of motionless resting, after the tears, as I waited for the pain to subside. Time lapsed and I conceded. *Okay, Lord! Your ways are far beyond me, and this pain you have allotted me has a purpose. Thank you for thinking of me and for planning what is best for me.* I settled for contentment.

Escaping the bathroom, I found momentary refuge in the fetal position, curled and silent upon my bed. I aimed to ignore the misery. I meditated on 2 Corinthians 4:16-18,

> "though outwardly we are wasting away … inwardly we are being renewed … our light and momentary troubles are achieving for us an eternal glory. So we fix our eyes not on what is seen, but on what is unseen. For what is seen is temporary, but what is unseen is eternal."

When my focus was on the cancer treatments, the hurts, the nagging painful side effects, I flew easily into the arms of despair. Faint in body, I felt immediately hopeless. This was the obvious. This was the focus on the seen. Yet, when I chose to fix my eyes on the unseen, all the work Jesus had done for me and through me during this trial, work even before I was born, I was filled with peaceful understanding. Inwardly, I was being renewed. I was made strong and mercy supported me. In looking for Jesus, I saw more and sang, "Open the Eyes of my Heart," literally, I wanted Jesus to open the eyes of my heart to see Him more clearly, more clearly, and even more clearly.

Musical choruses, along with images, and God's Word are hidden in my heart and I delight when they are called to the forefront of my mind in times of trouble; the light of God's glory shines.

Even still, as my humanness remained, I kept asking, *why did my God place me in these desperate circumstances?* The apostle Paul spoke of great pressures and declared in 2 Corinthians (1: 9b, 10b), "But this happened that we might not rely on ourselves, but on God, who raises the dead … On him we have set our hope that he will continue to deliver us."

Nearing the end of all my treatments, I was convinced that beyond all my hopelessness was a loving God who was refining me by the power of His omnipotent hand. I could not rely on myself, for I was weak, I was crushed, I was perplexed. I was down as low as I could go. In me, in my own vigor and strength, I had no hope. Outside my head knowledge, I was compelled to confront my heart knowledge. My heart was propelled like a rock in a sling, into the arms of God. I was in these desperate circumstances to rely on God, one large lesson in control. I had none, and He had it all. Deliverance would come, because Hope said so. Why? Verse 11b says, "Then many will give thanks, on (my) behalf, for the gracious favor granted (me) in answer to the prayers of many." God glories in delivering me for the praise of His people. *So, Praise Him! I am delivered.*

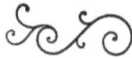

Offering Twenty Five:
Stick to What You Know

The end of the tunnel labeled treatment was here. Weakly I sat down in the sterile recliner for the last time, to receive my chemotherapy infusion. Many were congratulating me, smiles and pats on the back were given. I gave effort to be happy but I just couldn't seem to rise above the underlying apprehension.

Truthfully, I felt very much like the first phases of my cancer journey; fearful, doubtful, melancholy … and numb. Questions of the unknowns crept up and stole what should have been a joy-filled moment. Inwardly, I moaned and groaned, *what if this didn't really work? How long will I be cancer-free? Will my body heal completely? What if damage remains in my body? What if the cancer returns?*

Timely, Jeremiah 29:11 was the focus of the sermon the day before. "For I know the plans I have for you, declared the Lord, plans to prosper you and not harm you, plans to give you a hope and a future." God knew. God had plans for me. I knew that the hope and a future lay within the gift of salvation, yet, too, I had to believe and take claim in trusting that God also had a future set of

plans for me here on earth, beyond my last chemo
Monday.

Taking hold of that promise was the only way to
begin to erase my fears and apprehensions. This did not
come easily. Satan clearly did not want me to revel in the
joy of coming this far enduring the trial with success and
be looking to a future. The devil was on my back and
pressed down on me.

I fought depression during the last and worst days of
my chemo cycle. A dear friend sent me a dozen helium
balloons in bouquet fashion. Clipped to the string of
colorful ribbon were encouraging words calling me back
to Hope: "When you stick to what you know, the what-ifs
don't matter." Words simply said. Like a beam of sunshine
after the thunderstorm, these words cast a rainbow over
my day. What did I know? Of course, I knew a lot. How
could I ever have given the devil a foothold to press down
on me and steal my moment of joy and accomplishment
for having made it to the end of the tunnel?

It's all in the focus, just as I had realized many times
in this journey. All I had to do was to turn my eyes back
on Jesus, and look full in His wonderful face.

I looked back and fixed on what I learned and
experienced, firsthand, while my Heavenly Father held my
hand in this dark tunnel:

1. God gives assurance.

2. God stands with me.

3. God is in control, of everything.

4. God has a purpose in all He allows.

5. God is trustworthy.

6. God will never leave me.

7. God is beautiful.

8. God pours out His Grace, daily.

9. God sees me – in me, and through me.

10. God, the Father, holds my hand.

11. God answers prayer in ways we don't always expect.

12. God carries me when I cannot walk myself.

13. God is my Shepherd.

14. God is the Everlasting Arms.

15. God cares for me.

16. God never tires.

17. God has the power to do what I cannot do.

18. God's network is humongous.

19. God is my sustainer.

20. God works His compassion and mercy through His people.

21. God is Compassion.

22. God is Mercy.

23. God is my provider.

24. God never lets go of me.

25. God gave His only Son for me.

26. God is wonderful.

27. God is my Comforter.

28. God is my Strength.

29. God is my Peace.

30. God uses me, even in my weakness.

31. God is worthy of thanksgiving and praise.

32. God is patient with me.

33. God has a good plan for me.

34. God works in the hearts and lives of others watching me endure.

35. God is merciful.

36. God teaches me true love.

37. God has a sense of humor.

38. God sticks it out with me, even when I get complacent.

39. God is mysterious.

40. God makes me whole.

41. God sends messengers to uplift me.

42. God is steady.

43. God does what He says He'll do.

44. God delivers.

45. God does way more than I can ever imagine.

46. God is not idle.

47. God is MY God.

Stick to what I know. These words resonated deep in my heart of hearts. They plunged right into my soul. These 47 bullets listing *what I know* did not come from a book, a guide, or a how-to manual. These came from the front lines of my battle experience. When I pleaded in anxiousness, as I entered the dark tunnel a little over a year ago, and asked the Father, *You will be with me, right?* He was not kidding, when He said, "Trust me, I said I would be." God's love invaded the very fiber of my being and brought to life truths that I had read about, had known in my head, yet needed to have grafted into my heart. This journey was meant for my good. It was meant to change my heart and mold me to be more like Christ.

So, I say, *Stand down Satan! My God is on the move.*

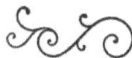

Offering Twenty Six:
A Greater Work than Healing

I have never been witness to the aftershocks of a large, devastating earthquake. I only imagine that a jolt of psychosomatic terror must immediately and fiercely ripple through the body with a chaser of adrenaline. Thoughts must surge wondering where to go, where to run, where to escape? All the while knowing there is no place to go, run, or escape. The ground violently rumbles, and the air fills with the heavy dust clouds of ruin and despair. If you are standing, I imagine you'd be immobile with disbelief of all that has happened. Dazed? Most assuredly, dazed and confused.

Dazed. That is the state that described me, that described my dear husband, as we drove down the highway on an errand one particular day after two routine doctor appointments, just a month after my last chemo treatment. Our eyes stared blankly ahead, our necks stiff with tension, breaths barely audible, and we were each wishing to go, run, and escape the news we had received earlier in the day. Just over a year later, on another fall day that displayed blue sky, a gentle breeze, and autumn colors marking the trees, we were experiencing the heaviness of untold dread. Unknowns again lay ahead, but this time we were weary. Could we really continue on?

Unlike the first telling, we did not pause to stop and find the comfortable and familiar place of each other's bodies and embrace. Instead, we sat still, in the aftermath of a quake, afraid to move for fear of upsetting the balance of a supporting beam and cause more destruction. Two routine appointments brought questions and more tests my way just barely one month out from the dark tunnel I had travelled with all the cancer treatments. A questionable mole, an enlarged thyroid, a spot on my mammogram, and a flattened cervix and atrophy of the vaginal walls brought many thoughts we did not want to entertain. This was the aftershock. It wasn't even definitive news that promised anything horrible. It was the upset, the blip, the possibility of horribleness that lurked in our weary hearts. Our balance was thrown.

Inevitably, the mole was removed, and the surgeon said, "It's probably nothing." These were not comforting words, as those same words echoed as a memory for me a year previous when another doctor told me, "It's probably nothing …," and that "nothing" turned out to be stage three cancer. Yep, I was feeling that psychosomatic terror ripple through my body. The thyroid ultrasound showed two growths and came with the recommendation that they be biopsied; the ground uncontrollably trembled beneath me.

Upon further examination of a second mammogram, the spot they saw previously was gone and I was told, "It might have been a fold of skin, this happens, don't worry, it was nothing." My heart wanted to leap for joy. I raised a thumbs-up at the technician who delivered the results and I smiled a stiff smile. It was those words that kept me from truly rejoicing in a piece of good news; *it is probably nothing*.

Good news was not familiar to me anymore and was harder to accept than I wanted to admit. Could I trust it? The cervix issue and the atrophy were side effects still raging from the radiation several months ago. Too much trauma to that area of my body, too much surgical trauma to my lower abdomen, rendered a swift path of deterioration. This was something. This was another low rumble deep in the ground. This would leave irreversible marks on the landscape of my recovery, much like the destruction caused by severe earthquakes. Some things cannot be replaced, fixed, or put back like they were.

I imagined myself in a better place by late fall of 2011. I imagined myself meandering across the green meadow, soaking up the warm sunshine and sweet life smells. I wanted to think I'd be singing, "Zip-a-dee-do-dah, Zip-a-dee-ay," with gleeful declarations of the beautiful day. I wanted a bluebird on my shoulder! I wanted that good ole Disney ending. But, it was clear that God was not finished with me and was directing my path out of the clear sunny meadow and into the shaded woods where it was dark. I was more like Snow White or Bambi, running and being forced into the scary woods.

Later that evening, when our errand was long over, I found my exhausted husband sitting on the bed with his elbows on his knees and his head hung low. His wide back was rounded and bearing weight it should not have to carry. He glanced at me sideways and I could see he needed to rest in the familiar place. I walked over to him and his upper back straightened. I stood before him wanting the same, and my arms ran gently across the expanse of his muscled back and his head pressed firmly against my abdomen. Finally we found the moment of breathing again, as we sighed and refueled, both relaying the commitment to stick it out – to travel this path together. God had to be our strength because each of us had none to offer for ourselves, let alone to each other.

We quietly prayed for healing. We earnestly begged for it. We asked for God's sustaining hand to carry us and provide for us all that we would need to persevere and do what pleased Him through this next jaunt on the path of unknowns. I knew that God was able to heal me and do far more than I could ever imagine (Ephesians 3:20).

Yet, I also knew that complete healing of my physical body might never come, even though He is able to heal me. I must submit to that understanding in order to gain Peace. I had to give way and trust that my Father, my Abba Father, was healing and doing an even greater work in my heart where the soul lives. He grew my faith in Him. As the words of an old hymn implore, God melted me, molded me, filled me, and used me. Yes, He might give me physical healing and He might not. He gave me assurance that I am His and that He will take care of me always because He is my Father and I am His child. Nothing can change that or take it away.

In this, I can praise God for being the total embodiment of Love itself and continually thank Him for the gifts in each day above ground. *Towdah* (!) for all He did for me this past year, and all He will continue to do.

This is my Song of Hope.

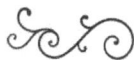

Offering Twenty Seven:
No Trust. No Peace.

The air was warm and the breeze silky as I sat on the rocky shore just before dawn, early September 2001. The sound of the crashing waves was both mesmerizing and calming. I felt the moist droplets of seawater mist upon my face. Suddenly and without warning, the first rays of daylight beamed up over the horizon. It was awesome! I felt such peace in that moment; it melted over me and rested for a while. This was a piece of time I wanted to bottle up and save. The dimness gave way to the sun as it rose and hung over the ocean, the light sparkled on the tips of movement upon the water. I loved our vacation at Long Beach, Maine. This was an understandable peace. I mean, who wouldn't have felt peace in that moment? Right? The peace stayed with me as I walked across the street to our cottage. Breakfast needed to be made for the eight hungry children now awake, and scurrying began to gather all up for another day at the beach. I felt peace slip off, bit by bit, like beads of water droplets dripping off a duck. I was happy, I was calm, but that peace that I felt oozing over me at dawns break was gone.

The Peace that surpasses all understanding is a

different breed of peace. This is the peace that I was claiming all year and that I wanted to continue to claim as I walked out and away from the tunnel. I know that peace is given to those who commit all their cares and worries to God with thanksgiving (Phil 4:7). It is conditional. Isaiah 26:3-4 tells me the way to have perfect peace; if I trust the Lord, forever, and keep my mind on Him, I will have perfect peace. No trust. No peace. It's definitely conditional. And I know that this brand of peace is one I need to face whatever God has for me in the future. Lasting; not fading.

Though I would never have chosen this trial, it was in this trial that I gained a greater vision of God and a closer walk with my Lord. I was given the gift of time to slow down and rest in the green pastures and still waters; He sustained me. I learned to trust more in God and less in myself. My mind was on Him and I mean to keep it that way. It is my hearts' desire.

Now I boldly ask that you would pray for me, and ask that God would reveal to me what work He has for me to do, and make me ready for it. May I continue to be used by and for Him, and glorify Him in all that I do, and enjoy it! That is my purpose. It is why I was created.

For you, dear reader, these plain and heartfelt words were written. May I boldly suggest that you too place your trust in the One who brought you into this world, who knew you before you were born, in the secret place. He will give you such joy, peace, and purpose in your life -- far above what you can imagine. And you too will be able to write your own multi-numbered bullet list of what you know about God. These truths will be interwoven into the very fibers of your heart and soul. Everything He did for me, He will do for you. Not in the same way, but in a way that is fitting to your unique design.

Be assured, God will be there for you when you are at your lowest.

Jesus loves you, my friend.

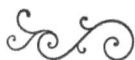

NOTES:

Chapter Four:
> *Fiddler on the Roof*. Dir. Norman Jewison. Perf. Topol,
> Norma Crane, Leonard Trey. DVD. MGM, 1971

Chapter Five:
> Green, Keith. "Oh Lord You're Beautiful." 1980. Birdwing
> Music.

Chapter Eight:
> Showalter, Anthony J. & Albright Hoffman, Elisha.
> "Leaning on the Everlasting Arms." Public Domain.

Chapter Ten:
> *Family Stone*. Dir. Michael London. Perf. Claire Danes,
> Diane Keaton, Rachel McAdams. DVD. Fox, 2000.

Chapter Eleven:
> Redman, Beth & Matt. "You Never Let Go." 2005.
> Thankyou Music.
>
> Watanabe, Esther. "With My Hands Lifted Up." 1970.
> Dawn Treader Music.

Chapter Twelve:
> *Pollyanna*. Dir. David Swift. Perf. Jane Wyman, Richard
> Egan, Karl Malden. DVD. Walt Disney, 1960.
>
> *Miracle on 34th Street*. "Dir." George Seaton. "Perf."
> Maureen O'Hara, John Payne, Edmund Gwenn. DVD.
> Twentieth Century Fox, 1947.

Chapter Sixteen:
> "The Ants Go Marching." Based on the Irish 1863 antiwar
> song, "When Johnny Comes Marching Home."

Chapter Eighteen:
> Dr. Seuss. *Green Eggs and Ham*. New York: Random
> House, Inc., 1960.

Chapter Nineteen:
New England Primer. *Now I Lay Me Down to Sleep*. WallBuilders, 1784 ed.

Sykes, Bessie & Seth. "Thank You Lord." New Spring. 1940.

Chapter Twenty:
Spafford, Horatio G. & Bliss, Philip Paul. "It is Well With My Soul." Public Domain.

Chapter Twenty One:
Grul, Daniel & Ezzy, John & McPherson, Steve. "Jesus, Lover of My Soul." Hillsong Music Publishing. 1992.

Chapter Twenty Two:
Kool and the Gang. "Celebration." Mercury Records, 1980.

Lewis, C.S. *The Chronicles of Narnia*. New York: Harper Collins Publishers, 1950.

Evans, Darrell. "Trading My Sorrows." Integrity's Hosanna! Music, 1998.

Founds, Rick. "Lord, I Lift Your Name on High." Maranatha Praise, Inc., 1989.

Kendrick, Graham. "Shine, Jesus, Shine." Make Way Music, 1987.

Chapter Twenty Four:
Baloche, Paul. "Open the Eyes of My Heart." Integrity's Hosanna! Music, 1997.

Chapter Twenty Five:
Song of the South. "Zip a Dee do Dah." Walt Disney Productions, 1946.

Chapter Twenty Six:
Iverson, Daniel. "Spirit of the Living God." Birdwing Music, 1935.

About the Author

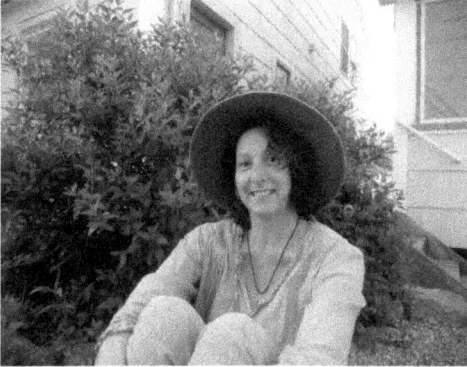

Sheryl Holmes

A daughter of the King, Sheryl Holmes enjoys a loving marriage with her husband of twenty-six years. She is a devoted mother of nine, currently home educating five of her children. Sheryl serves as an active member of Dwight Chapel's Christ Community Church, in Belchertown, Massachusetts.

Visit Sheryl on the Web at:

http://TowdahAlwaysaSongofHope.blogspot.com/

Coming Soon
From
Pix-N-Pens!

TOWDAH

A Cancer Survivor's Song of Hope

Companion

Devotional Bible Study

by

Sheryl Holmes and Phee Paradise

Watch our website and Facebook pages
for the release date.

**Look for other books
Published by**

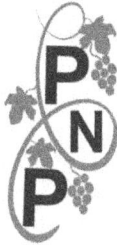

Pix-N-Pens Publishing

www.PixNPens.com

and

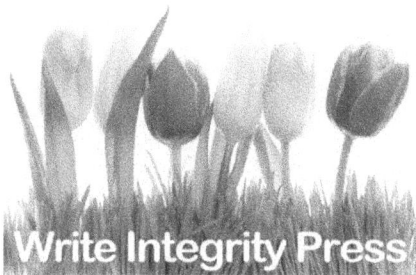

www.WriteIntegrity.com

www.ingramcontent.com/pod-product-compliance
Lightning Source LLC
Chambersburg PA
CBHW050133280326
41933CB00010B/1358